Dry Cupping for Beginners

A Step-By-Step Guide on
How to Enjoy All the Benefits of Dry Cupping
Therapy

Maggie Hansen

Table of Contents

Introduction

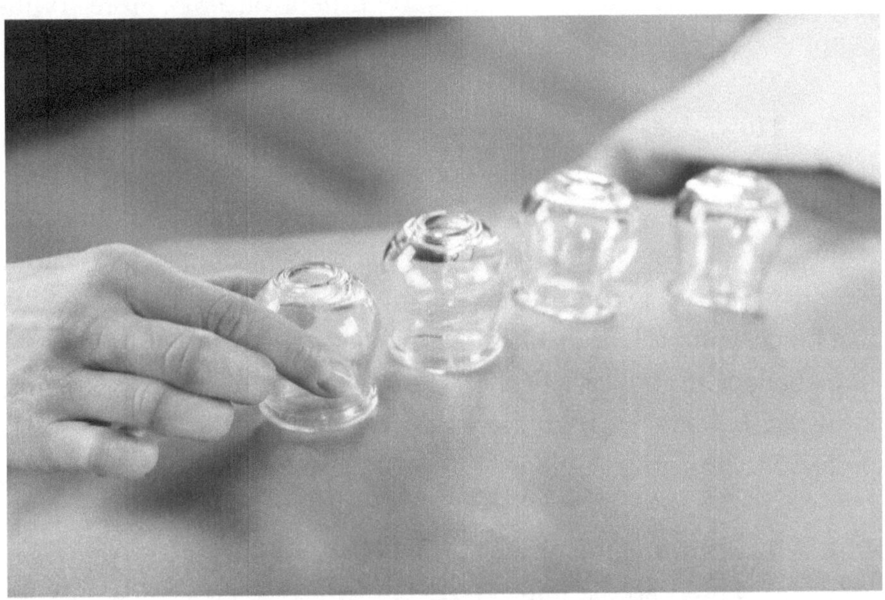

Healthcare has come a long way since the days of leeches, incense, and blood-letting. We created drugs and machines capable of treating all kinds of illnesses, improving quality of life, and extending our lifespans. However, researchers often find that ancient medical practices have value to them, and just because something existed a long time ago doesn't mean it should be dismissed.

Cupping appears in ancient civilizations such as China and Persia, and the technique has treated everything from sore muscles to chronic disease. By applying suction on certain points of the body, dry cupping draws healthy blood to an area and encourages healing and proper organ function. This book describes the various types of cupping used throughout history and when it's used today. Like many ancient medical techniques, there aren't a lot of scientific studies on the effectiveness of the treatment. Like acupuncture, many believe cupping is a pseudoscience, but there has been evidence that it does work. This book explores that evidence and the risks everyone should be aware of before trying cupping.

How does cupping work exactly? Therapists use glass, plastic, rubber, or silicone cups to create suction and treat headaches, stomach issues, skin problems, diabetes, fertility and menstrual pains, weight loss, foot pain, congestion, and more. You'll find descriptions of the techniques and images of the points that correspond to various health issues, as well as other treatments like changes in diet and Chinese herbs. People do try dry cupping at home, but for the best and safest results, a professional should perform treatment.

The information in this book is for educational purposes only and should not be interpreted as medical advice. It should not be seen as complete, exhaustive, or as a replacement for medical advice from a doctor or professional cupping therapist. If you are suffering from a health problem, you should seek out medical attention. Do not delay treatment or advice based on anything you read in this book. If you have more questions about dry cupping, contact a health professional.

C h a p t e r   1

DRY CUPPING 101

During the 2016 Olympics, viewers noticed odd circular bruises on the backs of swimmers like Michael Phelps. It turned out that the athletes had been receiving "cupping," an ancient therapy similar to acupuncture. Instead of needles, however, therapists use heated glass cups and suction on pressure points to encourage healing and promote wellness. When the heat from the cup creates a vacuum against the skin, it draws up non-circulating blood to the surface, along with toxins and other non-desirables. This allows healthy blood with oxygen and nutrients to circulate to the area. Swimmers and other athletes hoping for gold received the therapy to stretch their muscles and relieve soreness. While most American viewers were not familiar with cupping, it's actually used in more than 60 countries to treat everything from muscle pain to infertility.

Types Of Cupping

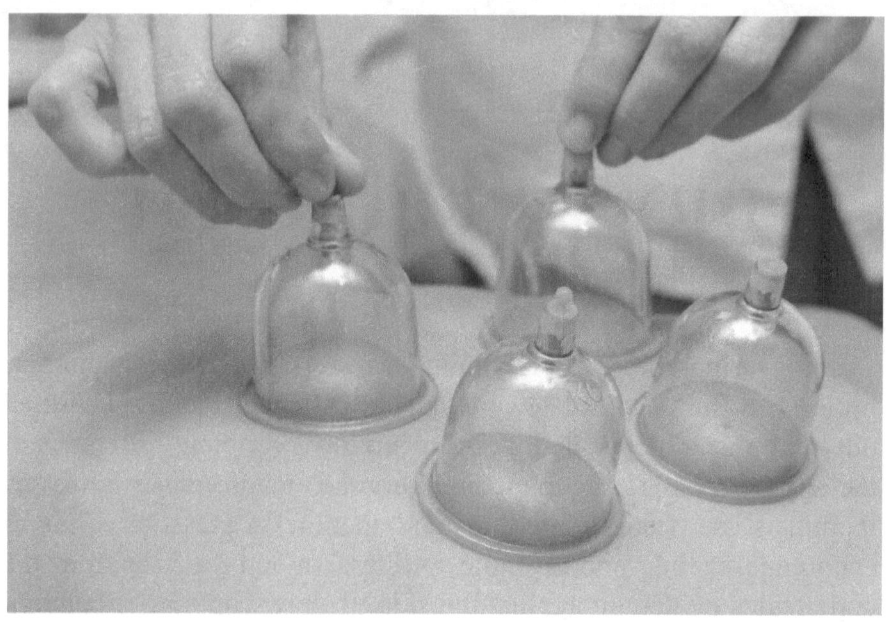

Technically, there are ten types of cupping, but they're all essentially variants of two main types: dry and wet cupping. Dry cupping is when a therapist puts a piece of lit cotton or paper into a glass, and lets the cup heat up. When warm, they put the glass against your skin and it creates a vacuum, pulling the skin up and increasing blood flow to that area.

Other dry cupping types

Within dry cupping, there are a few methods therapists will use, like *"massage"* cupping, which is when the cups are moved around. Oil is applied to the skin before the heated cup, so the glass glides more smoothly and adheres better. Because glass isn't flexible, therapists often use rubber or silicone cups instead. Unless otherwise specified, massaging in this book always refers to massage cupping.

Flash cupping often describes cupping done on the face. Suction is applied for a very short period of time - just a few seconds - and then removed. It's done several times during a session to stimulate stagnant blood, but it doesn't leave marks.

"Vacuum" cupping has also become popular in recent years and doesn't involve fire. You'll sometimes see vacuum cupping referred to simply as "dry cupping," with the traditional method labeled as "fire cupping." With vacuum cupping, the suction is generated by a suction cup. Sometimes therapists use a small hand pump, though cups that have a squeezable bulb on top are more convenient. Both forms of vacuum cupping let therapists control the amount of suction, which is trickier with glass. You can either massage with vacuum-cupping or retain the suction. In this book, you'll see retention occasionally referred to as "stationary" cupping to differentiate it from massage.

Herbal cupping

Herbal cupping combines cupping with traditional Chinese herbal medicine. Different herbs are used depending on the conditions the therapist wants to treat. Herbs are first boiled in water. The cup, which is usually bamboo, sits in the herbal water for 2-3 minutes. When time is up, the bamboo cups are drained, and then a folded wet towel is placed over the mouth. This reduces the temperature and creates steam inside the cup. The cup is then quickly placed on the body and pressed down for 30 seconds or so, until suction is created.

Wet cupping

Wet cupping (known as hijama in Arabic) looks a bit scarier than dry cupping, because it involves blood. The therapist performs normal cupping, leaving the cup on for 3 minutes. Once the cup is removed, the therapist makes a small cut in the spot and covers it with another clean cup (that's been prepped the same way as the first cup). Impure blood and toxins are drawn out of the incision. There's often quite a bit of blood, sometimes as much as ¼-⅓ of a gallon per session. After 5-10 minutes, the cups are carefully removed and the therapist disposes of the blood. The incisions are cleaned and dressed with bandages.

Less common cupping variations

Other cupping methods like needle cupping and water cupping have slight variations. For example, with needle cupping, acupuncture needles are used, with the needles actually left in place beneath a heated cup. Water cupping is rarely used anymore, and involves filling a cup ⅓ of the way with warm water. The burning cotton goes into the water, and then the therapists turns the glass over on to the patient's skin, ideally without spilling.

History

The history of cupping therapy begins in ancient China and Egypt, and spreads into Europe and eventually the Americas. Therapists used materials like animal horns instead of glass and plastic, and cupping often included a spiritual element. However, little else has changed - cupping has always served a medical purpose.

Ancient cupping

We can't say for sure what country created cupping, but China has been using it for thousands of years. The earliest records date back to 3,000 years ago when cupping was used to treat pulmonary tuberculosis. Ge Hong, an alchemist and herbalist who lived from 281-341 A.D., is credited with the saying, "Acupuncture and cupping, more than half of the ills cured." He described cupping in "A Handbook of Prescriptions for Emergencies." Using animal horns as cups, he drained pus from blisters.

During the Tang Dynasty, doctors used dry cupping to treat issues like stomach pain, headaches, and dizziness. It was often paired with other treatments like acupuncture. Other East Asian countries adopted cupping, and tools have been discovered in Vietnam, Japan, and Korea. Archaeologists have found cups made from pottery and bamboo.

Egypt developed cupping around the same time as China, with evidence appearing in hieroglyphic recordings as old as 3,500 B.C. The Ebers Papyrus, considered to be one of the oldest medical texts outside of Asia, proves Egyptians used cupping for medical reasons. During his travels, Hippocrates learned cupping and brought it back to Greece around 400 B.C.. He considered a good treatment for every disease.

Known as "al hijama," Islamic physicians practiced wet cupping almost exclusively. Originating from Persians, Arabs, and Turks, al hijama is described in the Quran. The prophet Muhammad advocated its use, calling it "the best of remedies." He used it for both physical and spiritual ailments.

In North America, there's evidence that cupping was practiced using buffalo horns, bones, and seashells. Little else is known about its history in this region.

Cupping in the modern era

Cupping has continued to be practiced as a traditional form of medicine. It was a common practice in Europe and the United States as late as the 1800's. In China, scientists collaborated with the Soviet Union and studied the effectiveness of cupping. The results led to all Chinese hospitals adopting cupping as an official therapy.

In the West, cupping has essentially disappeared from the general medical profession. Society shifted to the use of drugs, technology, and other treatments. Cupping gained a reputation as a method of the past, fraught with superstition, and Western scientists didn't give it much thought. It was still popular until the 1950's when it became relegated to practitioners of alternative medicine. It experienced a resurgence in 2014, when Gwyneth Paltrow appeared with the tell-tale marks on her back, and in 2016 when athletes used it during the Olympics. You'll also see cupping therapy offered in Finnish spas and saunas.

The science

Cupping has existed in many forms for thousands of years in Traditional Chinese Medicine (TCM) and the Middle East. That means it must work at least a little, right? However, you don't have to go far before you find a doctor saying it's all pseudoscience. Most doctors are iffy about cupping, with many being downright opposed to it. When it comes to the science, things get murky.

When someone is guilty of "pseudoscience," it means they're using "sciency" words to support an alternative treatment like cupping without actual hard data. The power of celebrity may be a factor in the therapy's trendiness, and as more people see high-profile athletes trying it, they'll start to follow suit. Consider Gwyneth Paltrow, who is arguably the queen of pseudoscience. She was cupping over 10 years ago. Now, with celebrities like Michael Phelps and Justin Bieber showing off their cupping marks, the therapy has attracted attention again. Based on what people have heard about cupping from these celebs - who are not scientists - they may think they're experiencing benefits that aren't actually linked.

There have been legitimate studies that link health benefits to cupping, so it isn't all hearsay. In 2015, the Journal of Traditional Chinese Medical Sciences published a report that said cupping therapy could be helpful for pain, acne, and facial paralysis. However, the study was also careful to point out that scientists can't draw a "firm conclusion" from the research. That's a common refrain in the medical community when it comes to cupping. This is because of the importance of the "randomized controlled trial," where participants are either given a placebo or the real thing, and no one knows which is which. However, unlike with pills, you can't "fake" cupping. Study participants who receive the cupping treatment immediately know, and it messes up the data.

Currently, the National Library of Medicine database has 300 studies on cupping and wet cupping, which is a tiny number considering how long cupping has been practiced. What all this really means is that we don't really know if cupping works. For years, Western doctors rolled their eyes at acupuncture, but now studies keep showing that it does offer a lot of benefits, whether it's a placebo or not. Will the same thing happen with cupping?

Risks

Wet cupping is riskier than dry cupping, because it involves cutting the skin. Infection is more likely, which makes it essential for patients to receive treatment *only* from a licensed professional. With dry cupping, the risks are significantly reduced, but sweating, soreness, and blood clots are possible.

In Australia, a medical journal revealed that between 2009 and 2016, 20 people were hospitalized after accidents involving cupping. In at least two of the cases, these injuries were caused by the fire, and not the actual cupping itself. In Hong Kong, however, a patient felt pain after the cups were placed on his skin. The therapist left, and unable to remove the cups himself, the patient had to wait 10 minutes. By then, he had severe blisters that took a month to heal. Good therapists *never* leave the room for long when cupping a patient, because it is important to monitor how they feel. As soon as he felt pain, the cups should have been removed from the patient. Traditional cupping (with fire) has also resulted in burns from heating the glass too much.

Both dry and vacuum cupping can cause inflammation and capillary rupture. Many doctors are concerned about the use of cupping to treat serious and terminal illnesses like cancer. Their belief is that the science just doesn't support cupping as a legitimate therapy option, and by forgoing the usual treatment, a person's disease could get worse and eventually cause their death.

When you shouldn't cup

Certain people shouldn't try cupping, and for safety, there are warning signs to watch out for. People with pacemakers should not try cupping, and if you are tired, hungry, or have a fever, you should also forgo the therapy. Pregnant women, those with skin allergies, those with a disease that can cause bleeding (hemophilia, thrombocytopenia, etc.), or people on a blood-thinning medication should avoid cupping. There are some exceptions, but it should *only* be attempted if a doctor says it's okay, and it should be performed by a professional. Other people advised to avoid cupping include the very young and the elderly.

When cupping, it should never be done on skin that's bruised, swollen, or ulcerated. If you have tender spots on your skin, it's okay to cup, but it should be for a shorter time and with less suction. In the case of fainting or feeling dizzy, the cups should be removed right away. To recover, drink lots of water and rest.

Health benefits

Uncertainty aside, users report lots of health benefits from cupping. It's used to relieve muscle pain all over the body, especially the back and neck, as well as stiff muscles. In a study from 2011, researchers found "suggestive evidence" that cupping can help manage pain. The reasons may be because cupping can increase endorphins and what are known as "heat-shock proteins." These help recycle old proteins, stabilize unruly proteins, and so on.

Another study (a randomized placebo controlled trial) showed that cupping can reduce pain in patients with fibromyalgia. Other pain issues cupping can help with include:

- Pain from arthritis
- Exercise-induced pain
- Foot pain

- Back pain
- Neck pain
- Shoulder pain
- Pain after giving birth

It's hard to pin down the health effects for certain, because there simply isn't enough research. Several studies indicate that dry cupping can help with nausea and anxiety, but a few studies aren't enough to prove anything. However, there have been connections between cupping and improved tendon-muscle flexibility, better regulation of the nervous system, a stronger immune system, stimulated metabolism, and detoxification.

People turn to dry cupping to treat nausea and vomiting; improve symptoms of asthma; improve facial paralysis caused by nerve damage; increase hair density; treat acne and scars; improve digestion; and treat symptoms of disease. In this book, you'll find cupping guides for a wide range of health conditions.

Summary points

- Cupping is an ancient tradition with roots in China and the Middle East.
- There are two main "styles" of dry cupping - with fire and without fire. Dry cupping without fire is commonly referred to as vacuum cupping.
- Massage cupping is when the cups are moved on the body, flash cupping is fast and doesn't leave marks, and regular cupping (stationary) cupping is when suction is retained on a specific point.
- There isn't enough research on dry cupping for professionals to say it's supported by science, and many doctors don't think it works.

- Cupping risks include blood clots, burns, and inflammation. Certain people should not receive cupping.
- Cupping therapists and patients report benefits from dry cupping such as relief from pain, a strengthened immune system, improved digestion, and more.

What You Need to Start Dry Cupping

Dry cupping tools are available on a variety of websites, including Amazon, so people often buy their own and perform the therapy at home. For the best results, you should go to a professional therapist, especially if you want to treat an illness. For sore muscles or other less serious health issues, dry cupping is relatively safe, provided you stick with vacuum cups and don't try traditional dry cupping with flame. As I mentioned in the medical disclaimer, the information in this book is intended for informational purposes and doesn't constitute actual medical advice.

Dry cupping supplies

What do you need for cupping? You have four options for cups: glass, plastic, rubber, and silicone. Glass is the traditional material, because it lets you use fire. Glass adheres really well to the skin, though you can't adjust the suction. In China, you'll find bamboo cups quite frequently, but because they can't be sterilized properly, professionals don't use them very often. They have narrow rims that often leave sore bruises, and it's very difficult to judge how strong the suction is, because you can't see inside the cup when it's on the body.

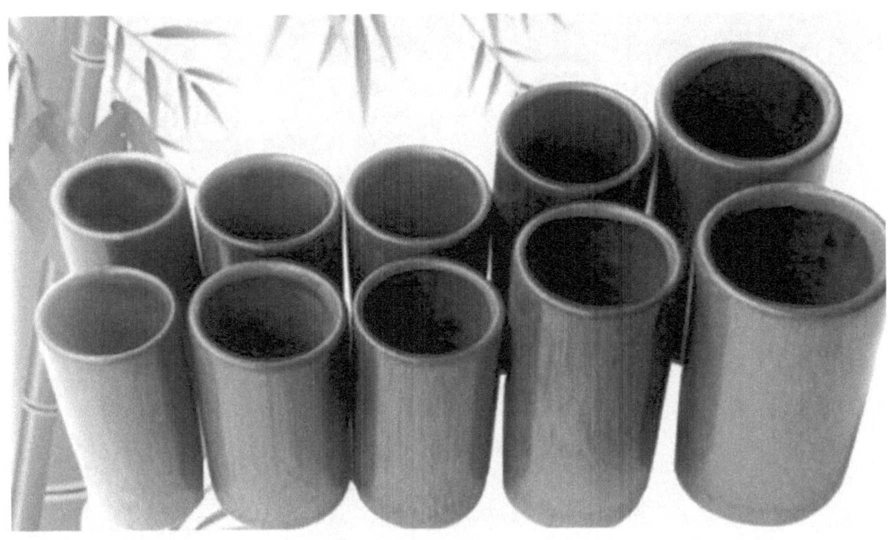

Plastic cups are currently the most popular for home-cuppers because they're affordable, they don't break, and you can adjust the suction easily with the use of a hand-pump. Hansol Medical Professional is a best-seller on Amazon (and top-rated), and comes with 17 plastic cups in different sizes and includes a hand pump.

Rubber cups are also available for low prices, and you can adjust the suction even easier by just squeezing. Unlike glass, they do not require the use of heat and won't break if you drop them. They are also very flexible and make gliding across the skin for a massage more convenient. Acucups make rubber cups, while Tai Chi Pump-n-Cups get rid of the hand pump so you just have to squeeze a rubber bulb to apply a vacuum seal.

For maximum safety, some people like to go with silicone. The food-grade stuff is what you'll find in professional clinics, so it's for-sure safe on the skin. Like plastic and rubber, silicone is flexible, easy to clean, and the suction can be easily adjusted. Lure Essentials makes a very popular 4-cup set. They also sell one designed in a smaller size for use on the face.

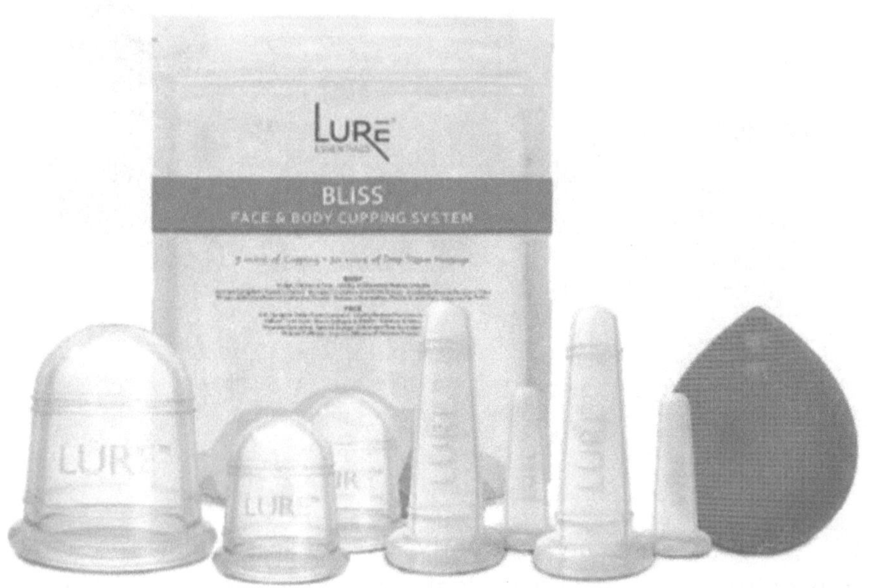

Wet cupping supplies

Wet cupping uses the same tools as dry cupping, although because blood is involved, you want to be sure that the cups are very high-quality and can be cleaned easily. That means bamboo cups are a really bad choice for most people. Glass, rubber, plastic, and silicone are all better options when it comes to ease-of-cleaning. A specific process is required: blood must be removed with hot water and soap, the cups disinfected with a high-level disinfectant, rinsed, and then dried. We'll get more into how to clean dry cupping supplies, since that's what this book focuses on.

In addition to cups, wet cupping uses a tool to make incisions in the skin, so stagnant blood can drain out of the body.

Plum Blossom needles are common. They look like slender, small hammers, but they have five spikes at the end, as you can see in the image on the next page. By tapping the needle on the skin, it makes small holes. Lancets and razor blades are used instead by some therapists.

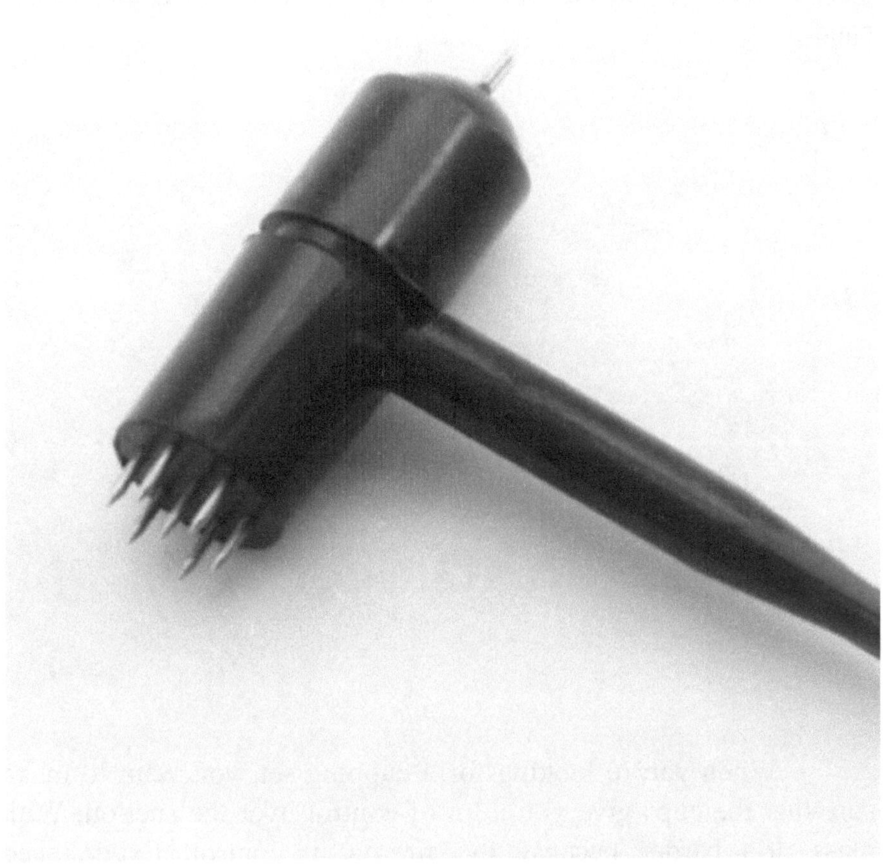

Dry cupping sets

When buying sets, you should have at least two different sizes. For beginners, a 2-ounce and 4-ounce are good choices. A set usually contains four cups in four sizes. Large cups are used on flat, muscular areas of the body like the chest, stomach, back, waist, thighs, and buttocks. Medium cups fit on the shoulders, neck, arms, and legs. The smallest sizes are used for facial cupping and for acupuncture points between joints and bones. For most cupping needs, a narrow mouth is preferable, though for boils and other treatments that involve skin issues, wider mouths are less painful. Below, you can see a plastic dry cupping set that uses a hand pump.

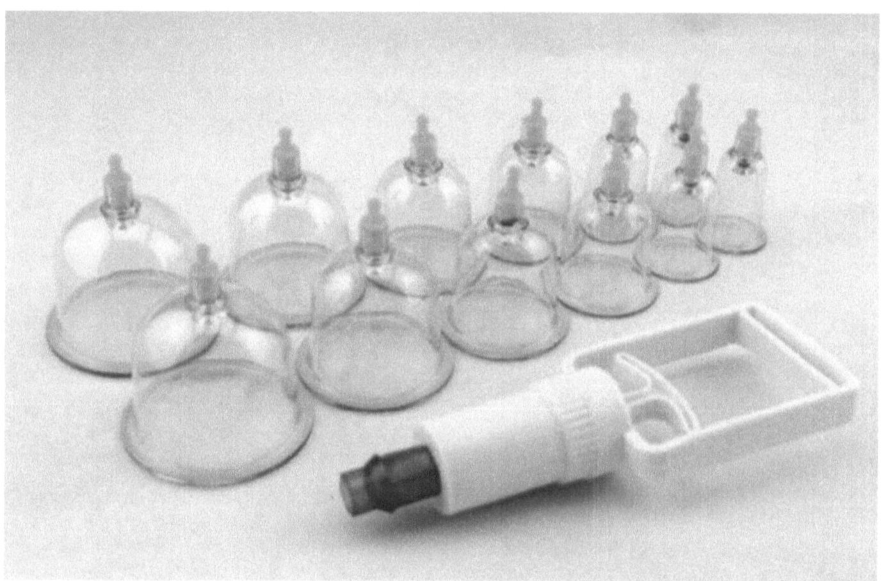

When you're looking for a cupping set, you want to make sure that the cups give you a lot of control over the suction. With glass, it's harder because the fire is in control. Experienced therapists will know how long to heat the cup and what level of suction they're getting, but the average person won't. Plastic cups with a hand pump, rubber, and silicone cups let *you* control the suction. A lot of people really like the hand pump, because it's very precise in a way just your hand and the bulb of other cups can't be.

Comfort is key when it comes to cupping, so pay attention to what the edge (or mouth) of the cup feels like. That's the part going right against your skin, so you want it to feel as smooth and comfortable as possible. Brands will even advertise their cup's smoothness as a selling point, so be on the lookout.

The last tip when choosing a cupping set is to actually try one out. Get an idea of how the cups feel in your hand, how they glide, and how to remove them. Like with any product, it's best to try out your options before committing.

Oils

Cupping often involves massage oil, which allows therapists to glide the cups around the body. What kinds are out there, and which are the best? You'll see terms like balms, lotion, cream, and oil. Balms aren't always convenient, because they need to be warmed and take longer to dissolve into the skin. Oils are the traditional choice, and you can find countless blends. If you're more interested in creating your own, you can use a combination of a "carrier" oil and one or more essential oils.

Carriers

"Carrier" oils are neutral and dilute essential oils to a safe degree. Popular carriers include coconut oil, sweet almond oil, and sesame seed oil. Coconut oil is one of the trendiest oils out there, and it's been used in massage for centuries. It can increase blood circulation, relief stiffness, and soften skin. Sweet almond oil is probably the mildest oil, and can be used on babies and children. When combined with essential oil (5 tablespoons of almond oil + 2 drops of essential oil), you get a blend that can reduce inflammation, relieve itchiness, and help with other skin conditions.

Sesame oil is the massage oil of choice for Ayurvedic therapists. Ayurveda is the oldest health philosophy in the world. Sesame oil benefits include increased joint flexibility, stronger nervous system, and healthier muscles. No matter which carrier oil you choose, you should always use it to dilute essential oils. For 1 teaspoon of carrier oil, 1 drop of essential oil is a good rule. This is described as a 1% solution.

Essential oils

There are tons of essential oils, but the best ones for massage will be aromatic, mild, and promote stress relief. These are four of the most popular:

Lavender - Versatile and fresh, lavender essential oil is one of the most common ingredients in massage blends. It promotes relaxation while also boosting stamina, and can help with breathing problems.

Eucalyptus - A natural pain reliever, eucalyptus oil is anti-inflammatory and excellent for treating muscle pain. Therapists use it on patients with tense muscles, headaches, and other chronic pain.

Peppermint - One of the stronger oils in terms of fragrance, peppermint is really good at cooling inflamed muscles and skin. Therapists use it for headaches, muscle spasms, and pulled or stretched muscles.

Grapefruit - A common ingredient in cellulite treatments, grapefruit encourages good circulation and softens the skin. It also has an amazing fragrance.

What do you need to start dry cupping? Here's a checklist:

- Cupping set
- Massage oil
- Tissues
- Towels
- A good skin cleanser
- Alcohol swabs
- Mild dish soap
- A low-level disinfectant
- Access to clean water
- Latex or surgical-rubber gloves (if there's a possibility of pus or blood)

Bruising

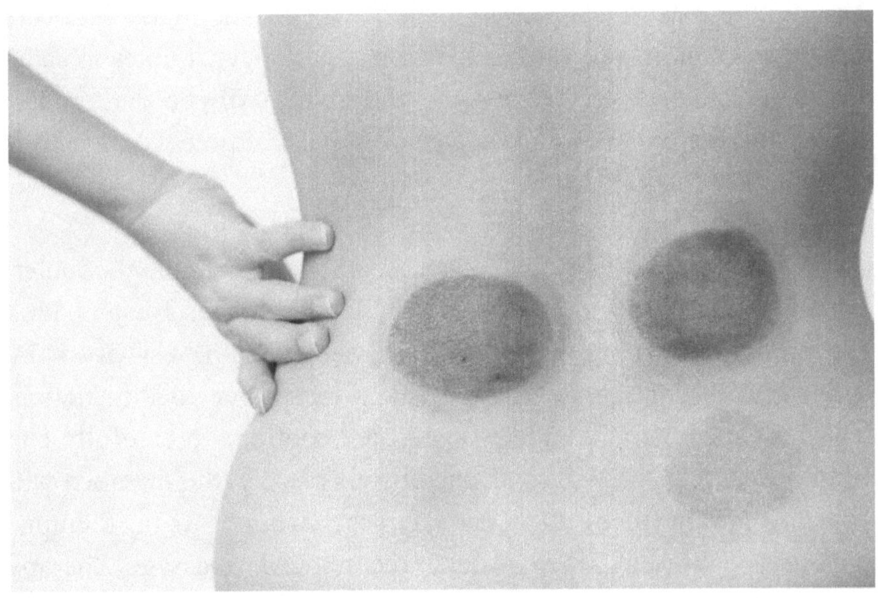

Cupping causes "bruising," but it isn't like receiving a normal bruise, which is caused by a traumatic impact and broken capillaries. With that kind of bruise, blood rushes to the area to heal the damage, resulting in the discoloration. With cupping, there's no breakage or trauma. The healthy blood is simply drawn to the area by the suction (instead of a trauma), and marks the skin.

You can expect marks to fade within a few days or two weeks. As you continue cupping sessions, the bruises become lighter each time. As you get healthier and the stagnation improves, the "bruise" will be light pink and can disappear as quickly as in a few minutes. With massage cupping, the bruises are less dramatic because the suction isn't held in one place for very long.

Bruising types

Therapists classify bruises by darkness. Bright red marks represent the least stagnation, while really dark marks indicate severe stagnation. The darker the mark, the longer it takes to fade. If the patient has very dark skin, the colors will be darker. For olive skin, the bruises might appear yellowish or greenish, which is normal.

There are a few other reactions therapists might encounter, which you can see in the chart on the next page. Blisters look especially concerning, and appear on people with very dry skin. Their bodies don't have enough fluids that move to the suction. They need to hydrate, and therapists can continue to carefully cup to improve fluid movement. If the blisters are big, the therapist will probably drain them and bandage the wound. If a therapist encounters blisters, they might recommend massage therapy instead of cupping. Depending on the severity of the bruising, it can be a sign of a more serious illness.

Purpura indicates there might be a serious health problem going on, so a good therapist will advise you to get checked out by your regular doctor, just in case. Black patches within the cupping mark tell the therapist you have really deep blood stagnation, and will require a lot of treatments. A white mark (following the first treatment) is believed to be the most concerning reaction to cupping, because it means no blood has rushed to the area.

Skin Reaction after Cupping

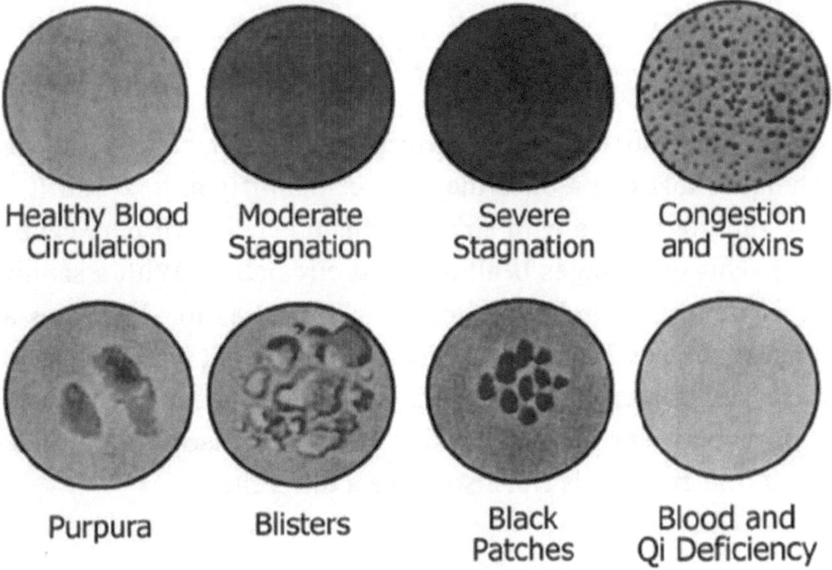

Here is a simplified list of the other types of bruising marks therapists see:

Purple/black marks - Stagnant blood/If marks don't disappear in a few days, more cupping needed

Purple marks with plaques - Plaques on skin appear as scaly white marks/Indicates stagnant blood and possible autoimmune issues

Light purple/blue marks with plaques - Stagnant blood, possible kidney deficiency

Scattered purple marks in different hues - Blood stagnation

Scattered bright red marks - Scattered marks surrounding point indicates problems with the organ closest to the cupping

How to get rid of bruises

If the appearance of bruises bother you, there are some techniques that can reduce them faster than if you just wait it out. First, rub the bruises with an anti-bruising cream (or pure cabbage juice). This encourages healthy blood circulation. With a sanitized hair comb and clean hands, "comb" the bruises for 2 minutes and then rest another 2 minutes. If you feel sore, wait to comb until the bruises feel better. After receiving a cupping treatment, be sure to drink more water. This hydration helps the marks fade quicker. Eating iron-rich foods can also make a difference.

Summary points

- There are four cup options: glass, plastic, rubber, and silicone. Plastic, rubber, and silicone allow for more flexibility and suction control.
- When looking for a dry cupping set, consider the size you want to use, the smoothness of the edge, if they're easy to clean, and how they feel when you're using them.

- Massage oils are necessary for massage cupping, and essential oils are very popular and come with added health benefits.
- Dry cupping causes dark marks referred to as "bruises." The color and texture of the mark gives the therapist information about the patient's health.

Complementary Treatments

Cupping can be performed as a standalone treatment, but it's often just one part of what a therapist educated in traditional medicine offers. There are five other ancient techniques you'll often see alongside cupping:

Acupuncture

Most cupping therapists also offer acupuncture. It originates in China and dates back 8,000 years ago, making it a much older therapy than cupping. Acupuncture is also meant to encourage a healthy, free flow of energy through the body to keep it healthy. By stimulating pressure points on the body using a very thin needle, a person can find relief from pain and healing from various illnesses.

Researchers have studied acupuncture for years, and in 2012, a large study came out that proved acupuncture to be an effective treatment for chronic pain. Using a group of 18,000 patients, the researchers learned that acupuncture functions as more than a placebo. Studies have also shown that acupuncture can be effective in reducing nausea.

Therapists might first perform cupping and then use acupuncture, or they might actually place needles and then put the cups over them and apply suction. The needle and suction work together, increasing the effectiveness of the therapy session.

Acupressure

Acupressure uses the same principles of acupuncture, but therapists just use their hands and elbows to apply pressure. Like acupuncture, the pressure removes blockages and allows a patient's life energy to flow freely. It's a good option for those wary about needles, and it can be safely done anywhere. Studies have shown that acupressure can reduce nausea in those undergoing chemotherapy. It also relaxed patients nervous about surgery.

Electroacupuncture

Electroacupuncture is exactly what it sounds like - acupuncture + electricity. A small current passes between pairs of acupuncture needles, stimulating the pressure point. To acupuncturists who use it, this boosts the needle's effectiveness and effects the nervous system. The goal is to release more endorphins into the bloodstream, enhancing the pain-relieving benefits of acupuncture. Electroacupuncture is used for all types of conditions. In this book, you'll see it referred to for weight loss.

Aromatherapy

The word "aromatherapy" doesn't appear in traditional Chinese medicine literature, but it's definitely used, and has been for thousands of years. Aromatherapy is defined as using extracted essences (essential oils) from aromatic plants to promote health. We discussed how essential oils are often massaged into the skin, but they can be inhaled as well through steam, and offer just as many benefits. Aromatherapy is used to encourage relaxation, and studies have shown that it could also reduce pain, anxiety, depression, and more. When you visit a massage therapist, odds are that they will have a diffuser, which turns water and an essential oil or blend into steam.

Chinese herbal medicine

Even more ancient than acupuncture, healing herbs have been studied for decades, and have proven effectiveness. They are used to supplement modern and traditional treatments. When you see a therapist who offers cupping and acupuncture, they are usually educated in herbs, too. The appropriate herbs are consumed a few times a day, and depending on what they're treating, you might use them for one month to a year.

There are two ways to consume herbs - in raw form or as supplements. Raw herbs are brewed like a tea for 30 minutes or so, but they're usually bitter and not especially pleasant. Most people prefer the herbs in pill form. Herbal medicines cost as little as $20-$30.

Types of herbs

Blends of herbs are more effective than single herbs, so you should look into traditional formulations. Here are eight of the most common ingredients in blends:

Ginseng - Helps treat health effects of menopause, PMS, high blood pressure, and erectile dysfunction. It's also used to boost energy levels, lung function, and brain power.

Lotus seed - Used to improve spleen and kidney function, and stop diarrhea. It has a naturally sweet taste that stimulates the appetite.

Ciwujia - Protects against premature aging and weight gain. It also helps with fatigue and regulates the endocrine system, nervous system, and cardiovascular system.

Black/red reishi mushrooms - Strengthens the immune system, improves effects of antioxidants, and can increase white blood cells. Both black and red reishis calm the body and can help with insomnia. It's also used for female sexual dysfunction.

Licorice root - Used for detoxifying and is a common ingredient in Chinese medicines because of its sweet taste. It can also treat common health problems like the cold, flu, depression, heartburn, and more.

Astragalus - One of the most ancient herbs used to improve digestion, metabolism, and the immune system. It can also prevent infections and treat wounds, though it can make other ailments like headaches worse.

Ma Huang - Also known as ephedra sinica, this herb treats congestion, seasonal allergies, asthma, and other similar health problems.

Ginkgo biloba - The oldest Chinese herb, it's used to treat lung and heart problems, chronic inflammation, and more. It's also a neuroprotective, which means it improves cognitive function.

Moxibustion

This treatment involves burning herbs to boost the effectiveness of acupuncture. It has warming and detoxifying effects. The "moxa," which means herb, is rolled into a ball and stuck on top of the acupuncture needles. It's lit on fire and sends heat and energy down the needle and into the pressure point. Moxibustion is used to help patients with arthritis, swollen joints, and fatigue. It's also used for pregnant women carrying babies in the breech position. You'll see it referenced a lot in the detailed cupping guides, though if you're cupping on yourself or someone else (and you're not a professional), just leave it out.

Gua sha

"Gua sha" translates into "rubbing congestion." The treatment is similar to cupping as it is used to encourage healthy blood flow. Using a tool with a smooth edge, like a Chinese soup spoon, the therapist rubs oiled skin to treat stiffness, tight muscles, pain, and more. In other Asian countries like Vietnam, "cao gio" is used instead. Also known as "coining," the skin is scraped with the edges of coins, and it often leaves marks that are mistaken as signs of physical abuse. Like acupuncture and cupping, research hasn't proven the effectiveness of Gua sha.

Talk to your doctor before trying alternative treatment

Most alternative treatment can be applied alongside traditional Western medicine, but you should always talk to your doctor first to make sure nothing counteracts with medications you might be taking. You should also not attempt alternative treatment in lieu of more accepted methods without a lot of personal research and consultations with experts. Just because something is natural, it doesn't mean it's good for you; and just because a treatment is ancient, it doesn't mean it will work for you.

Summary points

- Therapists usually offer other types of therapy along with dry cupping.
- Acupressure and acupuncture are older than cupping and have more scientific backing.
- Aromatherapy is using aromatic essential oils to promote good health.
- Chinese herbal medicine is an ancient tradition that harnesses the power of hundreds of herbs for every type of health problem.
- Moxibustion is when a rolled-up ball of herbs called a moxa is stuck on an acupuncture needle and burned. It's often part of an acupuncture session.
- Gua sha is when pressure is applied to specific points using a tool with a smooth edge in order to improve blood circulation.

- Always talk to a doctor before attempting an alternative treatment.

Chapter 4

How to Dry Cup

Cupping can treat a wide variety of health problems, and in this chapter, you'll learn just how to apply the treatment. The body, especially the front and back, are peppered with pressure points that correspond to important functions and organs. When stimulated through suction, you can encourage healthy blood flow and remove stagnation and toxins. Graphs are included to give you an idea of what pressure points line up with specific health problems like acne, headaches, diabetes, and so on. This chapter is designed for informational purposes only, and is not meant to replace professional medical advice. Unless otherwise stated, charts are from Cupping Resource.

Cupping strengths

Weak - The suction applied is very light and gentle. It only leaves a faint circle, not a full bruise mark. Weak cupping is applied for relaxation and improving blood flow. If you have a minor health problem like a cold, asthma, or sore throat, a therapist might stick with weak cupping. Because it isn't as taxing on the body, weak cupping might go on for a half hour.

Medium - The suction is a bit stronger, and light bruising is common. If you're generally healthy and being treated for headaches, stress, or a sports-related injury, medium cupping is common. In terms of time, a therapist might cup for 15 minutes.

Strong - This strong suction actually drains the qi (life force), so it's used to detoxify the body and treat more serious health problems. It leaves the darkest bruises.

What are pressure points?

The body is a series of connections that all work together. Pressure points are known as "meridians," or pathways through which life energy flows. In Traditional Chinese Medicine, this life energy is called "qi." When meridians become blocked or unbalanced, pain and other health problems arise. By applying pressure to the meridians, the body's ability to heal and function properly improves.

Pressure points are usually found in the body's natural indents, like the small hollow in the temple, between the collarbones, in the arch of the foot, and so on. The points frequently correspond to that area's source of pain, i.e. a headache is treated by applying pressure to areas of the head. However, points found on the opposite end or part of the body - called distal points - are often more effective at treating the problem. For example, there are distal points in the hand that treat pain in the foot, head, and back. Using distal points can be advantageous because it doesn't further aggravate the pain in the treated area, and it opens the whole channel of energy in the body. On the next page is a picture with the points' Chinese names:

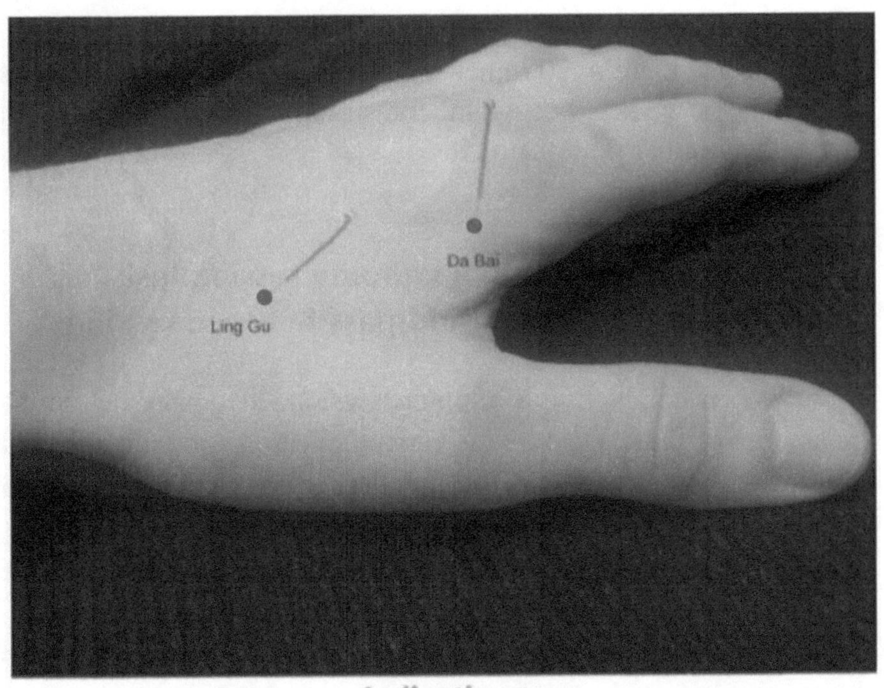

Indications

Ling Gu	Da Bai
• sciatica	• sciatica
• low back pain	• facial pain
• foot pain	• pediatric fever
• headache	• tonsillitis
• menstrual issues	• trigeminal neuralgia

In fact, all the body's pressure points have Chinese names and designations like P6 or GB21. The letters stand for the area of the body the pressure point affects- P is for "Pericardium" and GB is for "Gallbladder." You actually find GB21 in the shoulder. That's because in Traditional Chinese Medicine, the meridian of the gallbladder runs across the shoulders, back of the neck, top of the head, and the forehead. When that area gets tense, the gallbladder meridian is blocked and the gallbladder itself is affected.

In this book, you'll see the points named a few times, but to keep things as simple as possible, I've decided not to call attention to the names. Instead, you'll see them identified by dots. There are numbers on the charts, but I won't make reference to them often.

There are also a lot more pressure points in the body (after all, GB21 means there's 20 other points before it) than the ones labeled in the charts, but again, for simplicity's sake, you don't have to be familiar with them all.

How long should a cupping session last and how much time should pass between sessions?

When conducting a cupping session, therapists determine the amount of time based on the patient's health, strength, age, and physique. They also pay close attention to the skin's reaction to cupping. If after just 5 minutes of vacuum-cupping, the skin is bruising dark red or purple, they will likely end the session. If the therapist uses large cups, they generally keep the session short. Cupping on sensitive areas like the face, neck, and head is also shorter.

Patients receive cupping as often as 2-3 times a day if they're being treated for a cold or fever, while serious illnesses call for once-a-day cupping. The therapist does *not* cup in the same places, however, and won't until the bruises have faded. A treatment course lasts between 7-10 days.

Basic dry cupping (using fire)

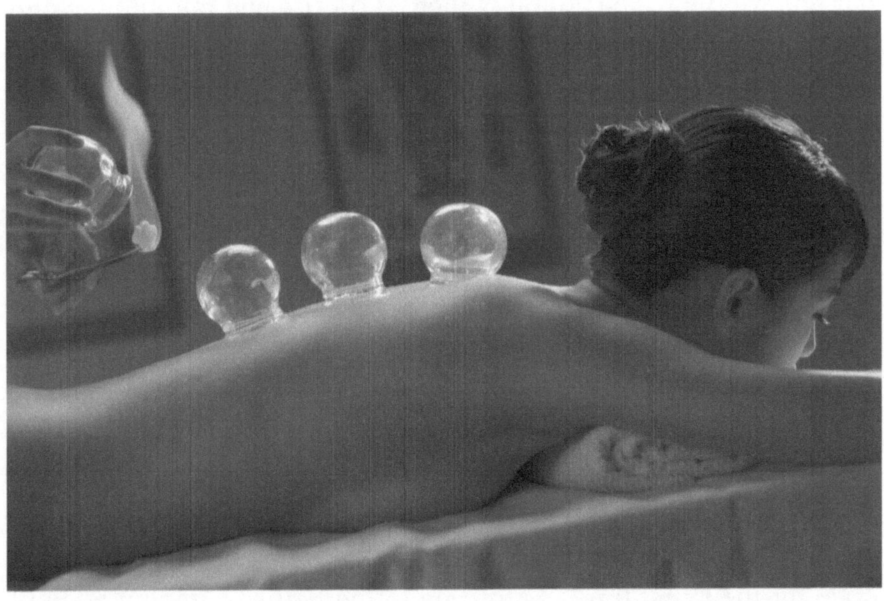

Before cupping, the person needs to be prepared. They should have clean skin free from makeup, lotion, or perfume. The skin also needs to be warmed, so they should take a warm bath or shower a few hours before. If that isn't possible or the skin has cooled, the therapist warms the skin with a towel or by rubbing them with clean hands. If the patient wants their back cupped, they should lie down on their stomach. If the neck or chest/stomach is being cupped, they lie on their back.

First, the therapist identifies where they're going to place the cups. If they are treating muscle soreness or injury, they go right where the affected area is and the areas surrounding. Fleshy areas on the back, stomach, legs, and arms are best; they won't cup where they feel a pulse or where there's an artery.

To begin the process, therapists saturate a cotton ball in rubbing alcohol (while it's held with long tweezers), so it's wet, but not dripping. The cotton is then lit on fire and put into the cup. The therapist holds it there for just 2-5 seconds, until the glass feels warm, but not hot. As soon as the glass is ready and they've removed the cotton, the therapist puts the cup over the person's skin. The heat vacuum creates the suction, and the glass sticks. The therapist wants the closest contact possible between the rim of the cup and the person's skin, so if there's hair there, the suction might fail. Using massage oil or even shaving the area can help the cup adhere.

There are a few ways to use cups - you can hold them on the person's body, remove them quickly, rotate them, move them around the body holding the suction, or even shake them. The standard time for beginners is 10 minutes, and most get 3-5 cups at once for their first time. According to the British Cupping Society, it's rare for anyone to get more than 5-7 cups during one session.

After 5-10 minutes, the therapist carefully removes the cups. If the person feels too uncomfortable or in pain, they will remove the glass sooner. If the suction is strong and/or the cup has been in place a while, the area may feel sore, so patients should move slowly and lie still for a while and relax. Like with acupuncture, you don't just get up and go after a session. Lie under a warm towel and take deep breaths.

In the meantime, the therapist cleans the cupped areas with alcohol swabs or a tissue. Rubbing the cupped areas can reduce soreness. If they used a lot of oil, they'll also clean this off. You shouldn't shower - your skin is still healing, and showering or bathing can disrupt that process. Wait a few hours.

Cleaning the cups is very important, because you'll be using them again and if they're dirty, it can cause health problems. Since dry cupping is performed over intact skin, they can be treated as "noncritical reusable medical devices." Wash with soap and water, and then disinfect with a low-level disinfectant, like a phenol, which is also used for intermediate-level, so you know you'll be safe. Be sure to wear gloves while disinfecting. You can find hospital-grade phenol on Amazon.

Once cleaned, you want to rinse the cup well with clean, clear water, so the disinfectant doesn't come into contact with anyone's skin. Dry well so no mold starts to grow, and then store in a cool, dry, clean space.

Basic vacuum cupping (no fire)

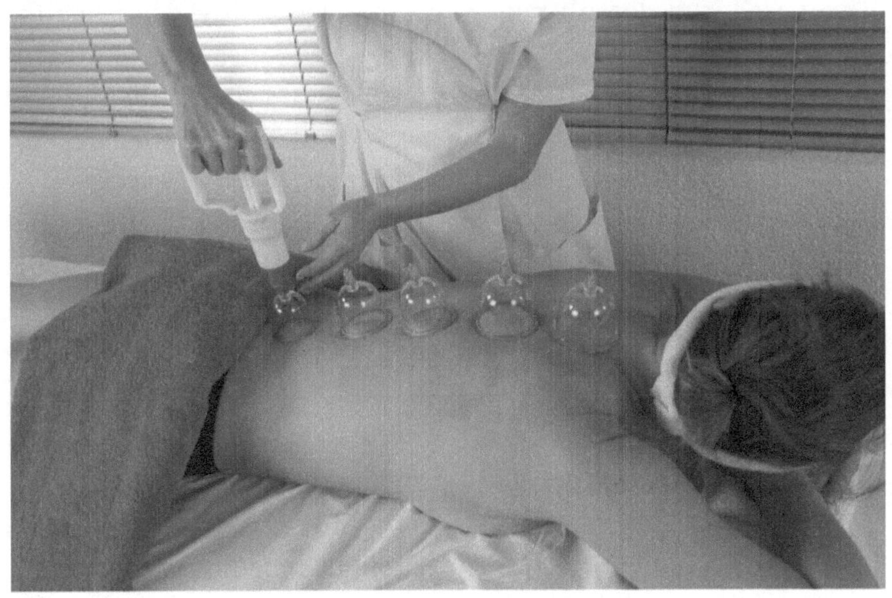

Not all therapists use fire when cupping, and if you want to try cupping at home, you should also forgo fire. Instead, you'll be vacuum-cupping, which requires plastic, rubber, or silicone cups. The body should be prepared in the same way as with traditional dry cupping.

When you've placed the cups on the target areas, use the pump to create suction. To do that, connect the cord to the cup. Pull on the gun handle, which draws air from the cup, creating the suction. Remove the connector, leaving the cup in place. If you aren't using a pump, the bulb on the cup itself controls the suction. Apply mild suction at first, which is best for beginners. Strong suctions can drain a person's life energy.

To remove the cups, simply squeeze the top slowly so the vacuum seal releases, and then remove it. Since you're at home, you can take as much time as you need to get the oil off your skin if you used it. It doesn't hurt you; some people just don't like the smell or the feel of it under their clothes. Mild dish soap and warm water, or a good skin cleanser can remove oil. Follow the proper cleaning procedures for the cups as described in the section above.

You just learned the basic process for dry cupping, but using cupping for specific conditions is a bit more involved. In the next chapter, you'll find detailed breakdowns of dry cupping for a wide variety of health issues, including headaches, the common cold, diabetes, and so on.

Can children receive cupping treatment?

One of the most common questions regarding cupping is if it can be done on kids. Today, more parents seek alternative treatment for their kids because of concerns about the ingredients found in medications. There are even cupping sets marketed towards kids with "kid-friendly" lotions scented like cookies and fruit.

While there's some debate within the cupping community about cupping on minors, most agree that it can be done safely. In a study in 2016, children ages 4-18 received abdominal cupping for constipation, and results showed it was as effective as the standard laxative therapy. As a general rule, cupping just should *not* be done on kids under four years of age. For kids 5-7, cupping should only be performed for 5 minutes, and then for ages 7-14 years old, 10 minutes is acceptable.

Another consideration to bear in mind: cupping causes bruises which may confuse some people. There have been cases where teachers and other parents believe a child is being abused. To prevent this misunderstanding, cup on skin that's covered by clothing, or let people know.

Summary points

- Cupping can be applied using different strengths, with the more serious conditions requiring stronger suction.
- Pressure points are pathways of life energy that connect all the organs and functions of the body. Applying suction to them taps into the body's ability to heal and support itself.
- Distal points, which open up channels of energy and are often located far from the direct source of the health problem, are most effective for treatment.
- When performing dry cupping with fire, the glass cup is heated and then placed on the body. After 10-15 minutes, the cups are removed. Cupped areas should be cleaned while the patient rests. Cleaning the cups is very important.

- Cupping without fire uses suction instead of heat to create the seal on the body. The process is otherwise the same - 10-15 minutes of treatment followed by rest and cleanup.
- Cupping is safe for children over the age of 4, though the treatment should be shortened to 5 minutes and then extended to 10 minutes for older kids.

Chapter 5

Cupping Guides

In this chapter, we'll get into the nitty-gritty of cupping and how to treat specific health conditions. Whether you're suffering from a headache, diabetes, or foot pain, dry cupping can help. You'll get a full rundown of the pressure points to target, whether you should use massage cupping or a stationary suction, and charts.

Treating headaches

A bad headache can derail anyone's day. There are four main types: sinus, tension, cluster, and migraine. Sinus headaches result from an allergic reaction, with the pain hitting the front of your head and sinus area. Many people think they're having a migraine when they're actually experiencing a sinus headache. Tension headaches often appear when you're stressed, and feel a dull ache (not a throb) all over your head. Your neck and shoulders might also feel sore.

Cluster headaches hit in a series, with each headache lasting between 15 minutes and 3 hours. As soon as one headache ends, the other begins. 1-4 per day is common, and it can go on for months. The pain is piercing and burning, centered around one side of the face or behind one eye. Men are 3 times more likely to get cluster headaches. Migraines, the most debilitating of headache types, appears as a deep pulsing inside one side of the head. Sufferers become sensitive to light and nauseated, with vomiting being common. Migraine headaches can go on for days at a time.

To treat headaches, therapists use facial cupping with movement to target the affected areas directly. The cups will therefore be small, very flexible, and made from rubber or silicone. Before placing the cups, it's common to apply essential oils that are known to relieve pain, like lavender and eucalyptus.

Cupping for sinus headaches: The target area is the forehead. Use up and down movements. You can also target the cheekbones and cup from the nose out towards the ears.

Cupping for tension headaches: Move up and down the forehead, and then glide the cups in little circles on the forehead.

Cupping for cluster headaches: Move the cup from the center of the forehead out to the outer edge of the eye. Cup both sides this way. You can also cup from the cheekbone towards the nose, and then from the nose out toward the cheekbone.

Cupping for migraine headaches: For migraines, you cup on the base of the neck, forehead, and cheekbones. Migraines are caused by a reduction of blood supply to the brain. During a migraine, muscles spasm at the base of the skull, restricting the blood flow. To offset, the blood vessels in the brain expand, creating painful nerve tension in your head. When you receive cupping on the neck, forehead, and cheekbones, the muscles relax as the suction of the cups draws more blood to the area. Move the cup up and down over the forehead, and side to side below the eyes. The cup can also move out from the nose to the cheekbones. You can also receive cupping on the neck and shoulders.

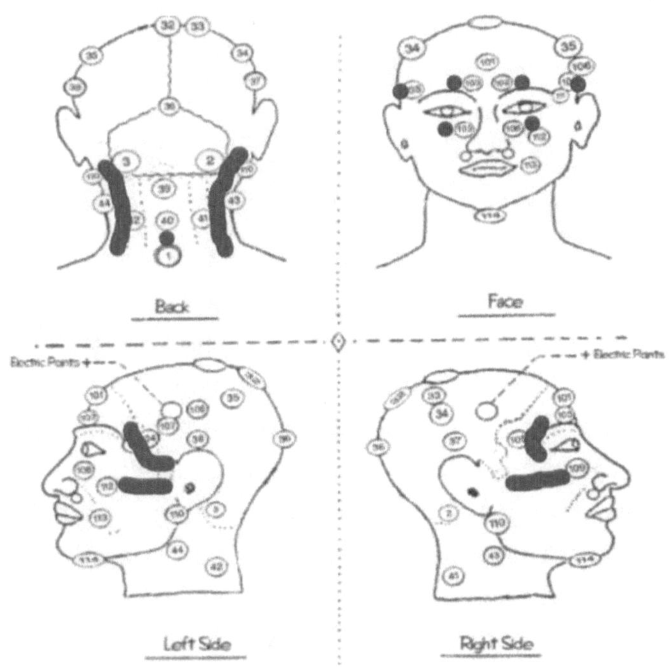

Cupping for general-stress headaches: Regardless of your headache type, cupping on the neck and shoulders can help. Place the suction cup behind the ear and then move down over the neck and out to the shoulders. This improves circulation. There is also a point on the hand known to treat headaches. It's called "Nei Guan," or simply P6.

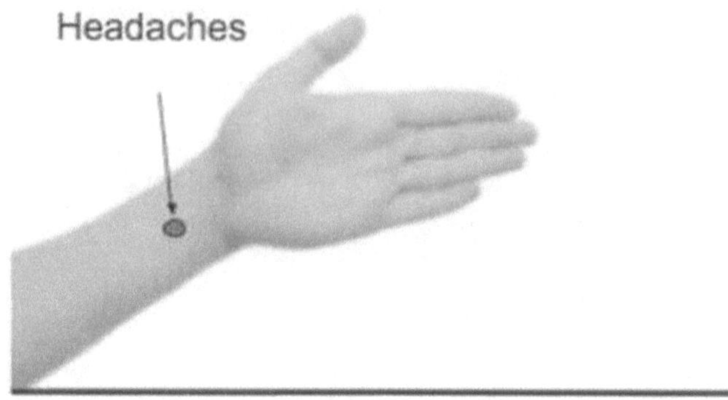

Other headache treatments: Because headaches can be a sign of another health condition, additional treatment should be decided based on what that condition is. In general, avoiding spicy food, smoking, alcohol, coffee, strong tea, and sugar can help. It's also important to get plenty of quality sleep and reduce stress. Herbs such as Chinese wild ginger, chamomile, basil, and lavender can help. Depending on what type of headache you have, therapists will identify what herb is most effective.

Nosebleeds

Frequent and heavy nosebleeds are a cause for concern. While everyone gets a nosebleed now and then, more regular ones can be caused by hypertension, severe allergies, an infectious disease, or a bleeding disease. According to Traditional Chinese Medicine, nosebleeds are caused by overheated blood in the lung, stomach, or liver-kidney meridian. It could also be because of a spleen deficiency.

When cupping for nosebleeds, there are a variety of points that therapists might use, depending on what they believe the problem is. Cupping can be done on the face right next to the nostrils and on the back of the head. There's also a point on top of the head. For the hand, there are two points: one is on the outer edge of the thumb right by the nail, and the other is on the index finger close to the lower knuckle. Because these points are so small, the therapist might use acupressure in place of cupping. On the legs, there are points by the ankle and on the inner edge of the lower calf on the front of the leg. The little point on the foot is on the top of the foot between the bones of the big toe and index toe.

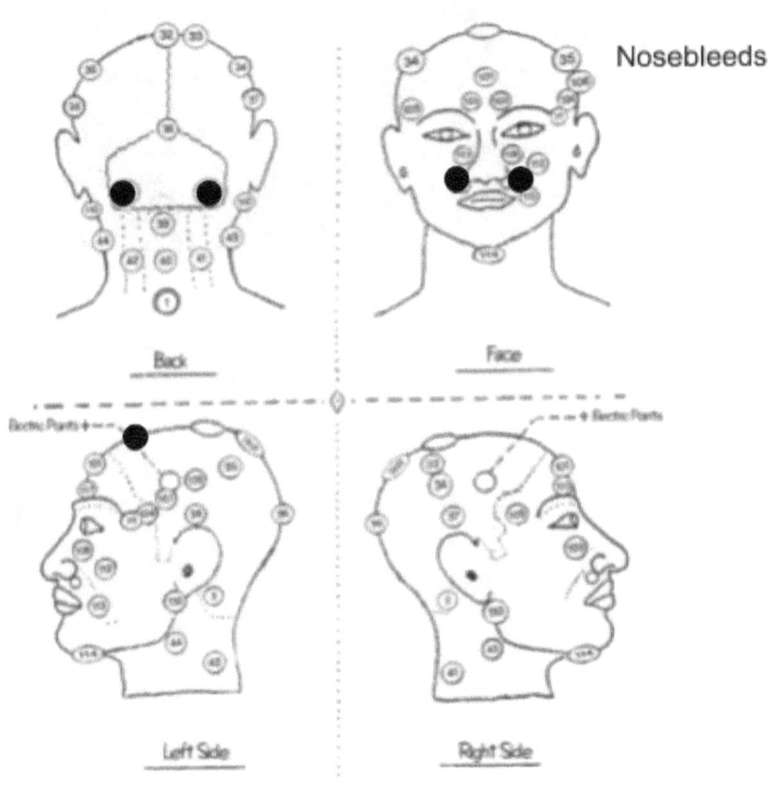

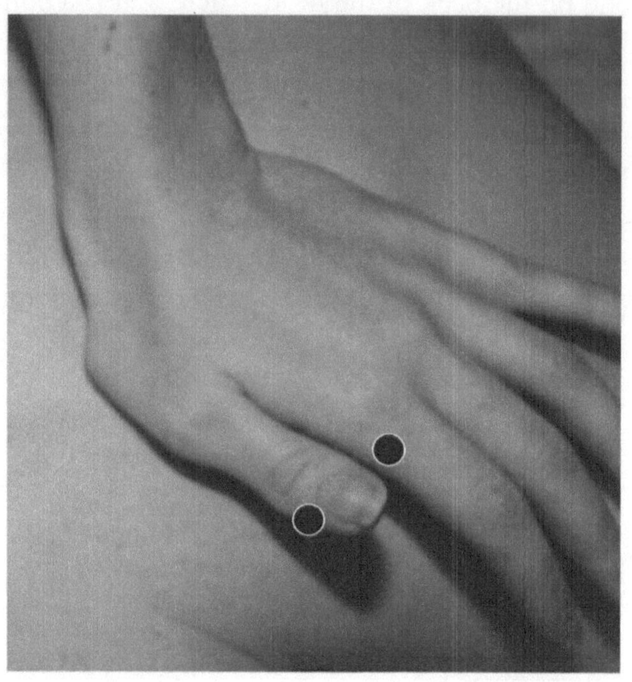

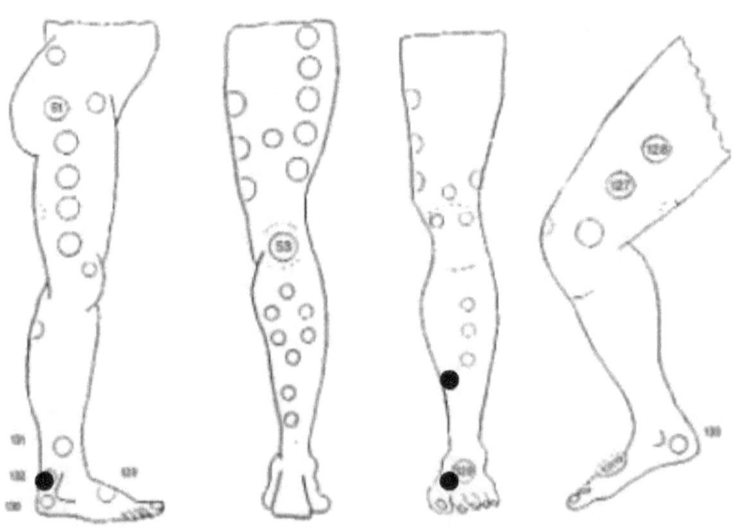

Other treatments for nosebleeds

To prevent nosebleeds, you should make sure that the air in your home is moist. Get a humidifier for your bedroom. You can also elevate your head with one or two pillows. In terms of diet, dark leafy veggies provide Vitamin K, which helps blood clot properly, while citrus fruit and Vitamin C strengthen blood cells and help the body form collagen. Avoid alcohol, smoking, and drugs that thin the blood. Because nosebleeds are caused by overheated blood, cooling herbs are best. These include couch grass, field thistle, peppermint, and chrysanthemum.

Anxiety + depression

Anxiety is a common condition in our hectic society. It manifests as nervousness, fear, headaches, insomnia, and so on. There are pressure points on the wrist, foot, and back. The point on the wrist is parallel to the little finger. Rub for a few minutes to warm the area and then apply suction for 5-10 minutes. Repeat on the other hand. The point on the foot is found on top, between the bones of the big toe and the toe next to it. On the back, apply suction below the neck and between the shoulder blades on both sides of the spine.

Depression is one of the most common mental conditions in the US, and medications often come with a lot of side effects. For mild to moderate depression, people turn to dietary treatments and cupping. For depression, the points are the same as anxiety, with a few extras. The therapist will also apply moving cupping instead of stationary. Move the cups on the points back and forth, up and down. After the massage, suction can be applied for 5 minutes.

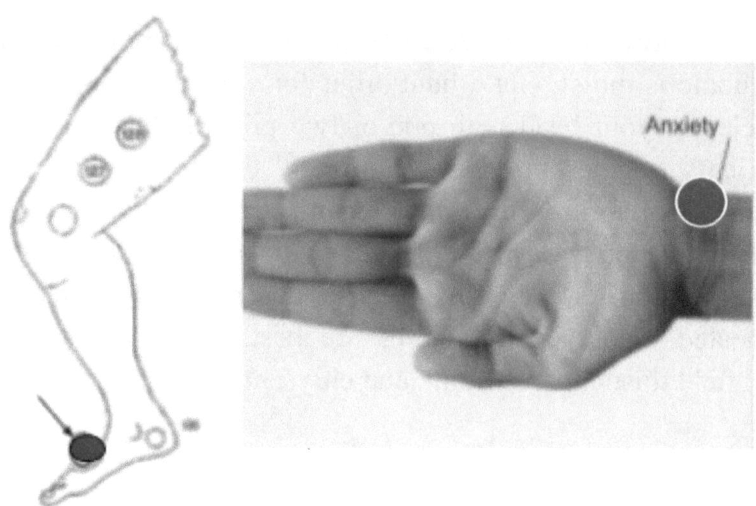

Anxiety

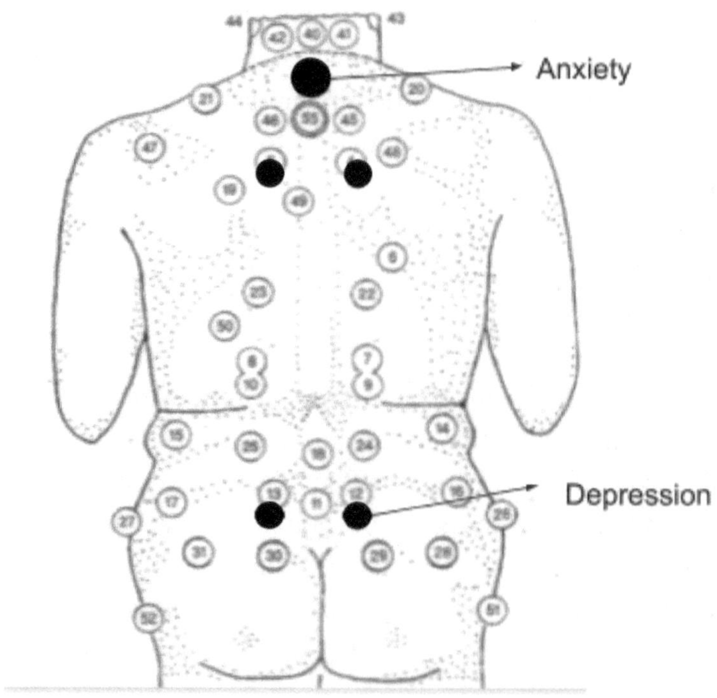

Anxiety
Depression

Other treatments for anxiety and depression

Anxiety can be treated by emotional regulation and directing nervous energy towards productive hobbies and interests. Consider meditation and other relaxing habits. For depression, a diet rich in vitamin B and amino acids can help. It's also important to surround oneself with a community that's supportive and loving. Talk therapy is also very effective.

Before medication, people used herbs. Herb blends brewed in teas are very popular since they are easy to make and soothing. In Traditional Chinese Medicine, there are substances that treat nervousness, anxiety, depression, and the symptoms of these conditions. Traditional Chinese Medicine always links issues back to the organs, so the herb formulations align with the liver, heart, and so on. Ingredients include white peony root, ginger, and licorice. Some even include materials like powdered fossils and oyster shells, which contain calcium and heavy metals. These were meant just for the short-term, because long-term they can damage the body.

Insomnia

When you don't get enough sleep, your whole body (and mind) suffers. Insomnia is often accompanied by headaches, fatigue, and dizziness. It can be caused by stress, nutritional problems, pain, neurological problems, and so on. To treat insomnia through cupping, therapists focus on the forearm and back. For the arm, find the point on the inside of your wrist parallel to the pinky finger. Massage with the thumb for a while to warm up the area. With the smallest cup you have, apply vacuum suction for 5-10 minutes.

For the back, you're going to be massaging points (with a cup) alongside the spine. There's a meridian there that flows down all the way to the foot. For insomnia, therapists want to pay special attention to those pressure points. They may choose to apply stationary cupping on them for 5 minutes after the cupping massage.

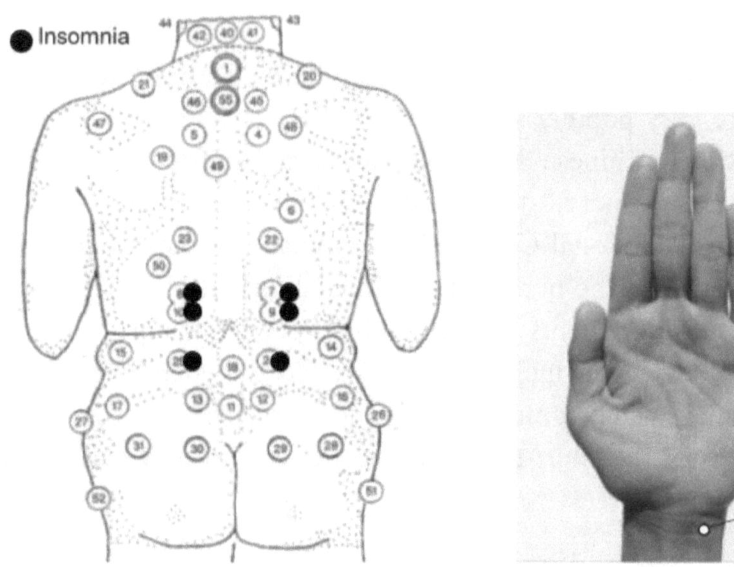

Other insomnia treatments

Using Traditional Chinese Medicine, you can also treat insomnia with diet and other healthy habits. Therapists might recommend eating porridge made with food that boosts qi and blood circulation, such as red dates and black sesame seeds. Before going to bed, drinking a glass of warm milk could also help. At the same time, try soaking your feet in hot water until your forehead just begins to sweat. This encourages good blood circulation, which promotes sleep.

Begin "winding down" an hour or so before you need to be in bed; doing relaxing activities tells your body it's time to sleep. Sleep in complete darkness, without electronics, so the body can produce melatonin, a natural sleep aid. Light disrupts this process. Avoid strong tea, smoking, and coffee while undergoing treatment.

For herbs, therapists choose them based on what they think is causing insomnia. It could be a deficiency in the heart or liver, so the herbs will differ slightly. Calming herbal teas are a good addition to an evening routine. Albizia flower tea helps relieve stress, depression, and chest tightness. Lotus plumule tea, which is often made with licorice root, can also help, as can teas made from red dates and acorus.

Treating stomach and digestion issues

Digestive issues are some of the most common health problems that people face. Stress and anxiety are closely-linked to stomach pains, constipation, bloating, and more. In Traditional Chinese Medicine, all foods are classified by temperature and flavor: hot, cold, spicy, sweet, sour, and pungent. These all affect the body in different ways, and to be healthy, one must have the right balance. When you don't eat properly, it causes weak "digestive fire," leading to problems like indigestion, constipation, etc. Adopting a balanced diet is essential to regaining good health, and dry cupping can play a helpful role, too.

Dry cupping can help jumpstart healthy qi movement again and stoke the body's digestive fire. The cupping occurs right on the problem areas, like the stomach, navel, over the bladder, and around the kidneys. Applying suction stimulates the organs so they can perform their functions properly.

To cup the abdomen, rub oil on clean skin and then apply the cup and suction. Slide the cup around the stomach in a clockwise motion. The patient should feel stretching, but no pain. You can also vacuum-cup around the belly button, leaving the cups for the standard 5-10 minutes. Cupping in this area increases the flow of digestive juices. If you're experiencing diarrhea, belly-button cupping may help. Moxibustion is typically performed after cupping for 3-5 minutes. You can see the points below in dark.

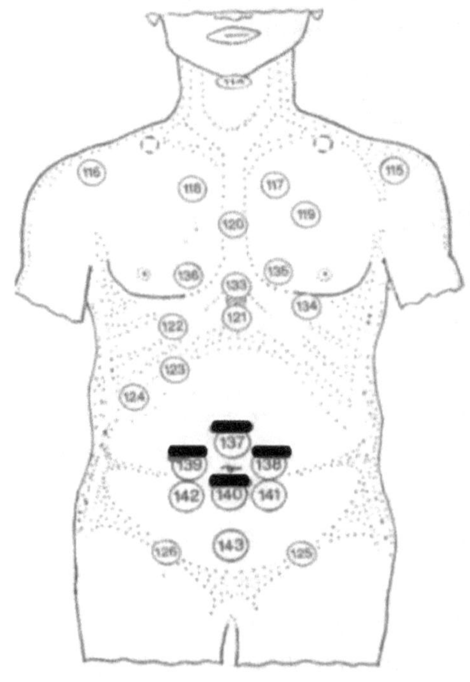

Acid reflux

Acid reflux occurs when the acidic fluid from the gastric intestine goes up into the esophagus. This causes heartburn and it can wear away the lining of the esophagus. It can also lead to acid reflux disease, which is considered a chronic condition. Acid reflux can be caused by stomach abnormalities, pregnancy, smoking, and certain foods, especially spicy ones.

According to Traditional Chinese Medicine, energy imbalances cause acid reflux. Energy stagnates in the liver and combines with cool moisture from the spleen, leading to excess heat and moisture in the stomach. The acid shoots up into the esophagus as a result.

Cupping can be performed on the chest, between the breastbone and belly button, as well as on the arch of the foot and on the back of the head. Why in such different places? Those are where the meridians flow, and opening up the whole channel of energy is extremely effective in treating the root of the problem. Cupping on the head should be short - just 1 or 2 minutes - and light suction should be applied for the first time.

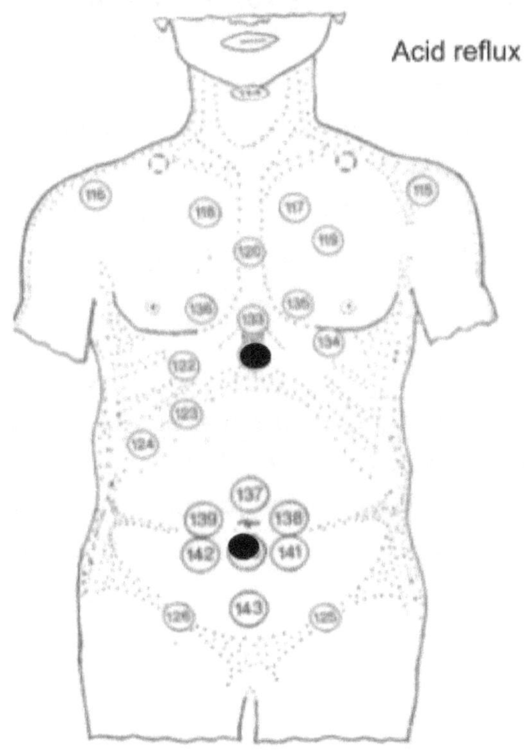

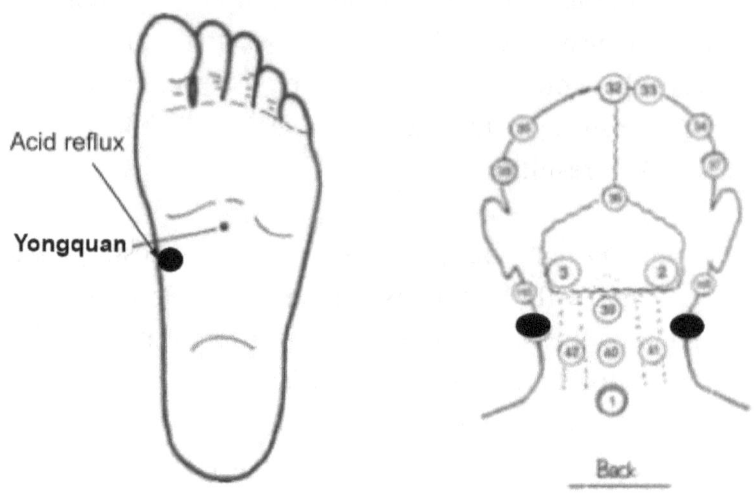

Other treatments for stomach issues

Stomachaches can be caused by a number of factors, so pay attention to what you're eating. Avoid raw, cold food, as well as food that's overly sour and spicy. Adopt a consistent eating schedule. Stomachaches can also be caused by anxiety, so reduce the stress in your life. Ginger is used frequently to treat stomach pain.

If you suffer from diarrhea, a change in diet can help significantly. Soft rice soup, weak tea, and juice are all good. If you have chronic diarrhea, yams, lotus root starch, and water prevent dehydration. To prevent diarrhea, avoid cool food and drink. A therapist might also use herbs like peony, ginger, tangerine, and licorice.

If constipation is the problem, be wary of laxatives, as they can be too harsh on the body. Eat more fiber-rich foods, like apples, bananas, grapes, red dates, and vegetables. Also be sure to drink plenty of water and get some exercise. Herbs for constipation include black sesame seeds and rhubarb root.

To treat acid reflux, avoid spicy and fatty foods. Drinking alcohol can also trigger acid reflux, so cut down. You should also avoid eating right before bedtime or before lying down. Herbs like yarrow, gold thread, and barberry encourage drying, while slippery elm and marshmallow root protect against the acid.

Problems with menstruation

Period cramps are one of the most common problems for women and can cause other issues like headaches, back pain, and vomiting. Known scientifically as "dysmenorrhea," cramping is associated with high levels of "prostaglandins," which are compounds released during the breakdown of the uterine lining. Prostaglandins cause the uterus muscles to contract, causing pain. Other chemicals in the body may play a role, too.

Cupping can reduce the number of prostaglandins. At the same time, it can encourage the production of endorphins, the body's natural painkiller, and relax the patient. Abdominal cupping, which was described in the section on stomach issues, can be performed. A therapist can also use cupping on the areas marked on the graph on the next page in dark. A therapist should *not* use cups on a patient currently suffering from cramps; it can be done at any other time during the menstrual cycle and will be beneficial.

Another common issue women face is abnormally-heavy bleeding. In a study about the effects of dry cupping and the effectiveness of cupping, researchers put two large cups right below the breasts of patients for 15 minutes. Results found that bleeding was reduced, but the study acknowledges that more research should be done.

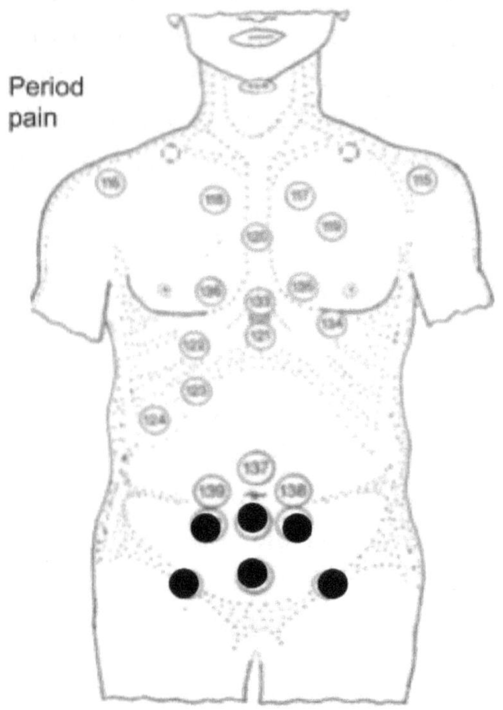

Other treatments for painful periods

When period cramps are very painful, a woman can drink liquids known to increase qi, such as red ginger or red raspberry tea, which strengthens the uterine tissue. Peppermint tea may also help. For food, fish oil and foods high in B1 can relieve pain. While having your period, you should also avoid intense exercise or sex, and avoid getting too cold, especially at night. Some light exercise can help though, since it releases pain-relieving endorphins. Stay hydrated.

In Traditional Chinese Medicine, there's a formula designed to reduce cramping. It's made from ingredients like peony root and bark, safflower, and Dong Quai root. Orange peel, silk tree, red clover, and angelica can also relieve pain.

Irregular periods

Another very common issue women face is irregular periods. A "regular" period should occur every 28-30 days and last between 3-7 days. The most important indicator of a regular period is that the same number of days pass between each period. Irregular periods are marked by general symptoms like cramps and bloating at random times during the month, and the time between periods isn't the same. Causes include certain medications, intense and frequent exercise, eating disorders, hormonal issues, and stress.

Cupping is usually performed 3-5 days before menstruation (though if the woman doesn't know when the period will be, that can be tricky) and also 2 days after bleeding stops. There are two groups of points, so cupping will be performed on one group one day, and then the second group the next day. Points on the leg and foot should be massaged first. Moxibustion is usually performed after the cupping for 3-5 minutes.

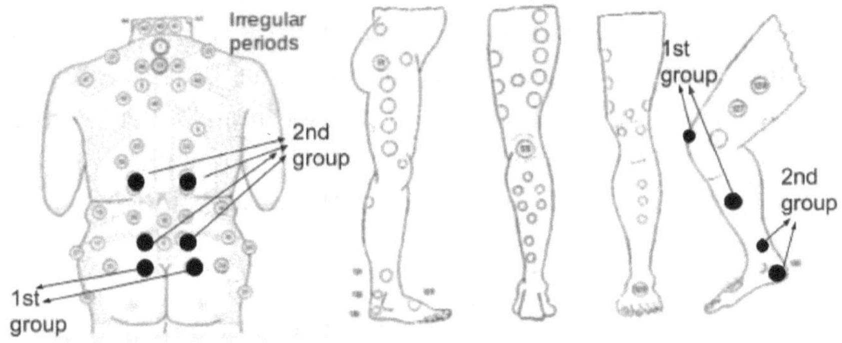

The first group of points can be found on top of the buttocks, on the inner edge of the shinbone parallel to the calf, and close to the knee, when it's bent. Apply vacuum cupping for 10-15 minutes, then perform moxibustion. For the second group, the points are on the middle back and on the lower lumbar, above the first points. You'll be massaging with the cups in this area, and then the therapist may choose to stationary cup afterwards. You can also cup on the heel and above the ankle.

Other treatments for irregular periods

A change in diet can help regulate your period. Eat more mutton, freshwater shrimp, red dates, black beans, and walnuts. Any food high in iron is a good idea, though you should avoid raw, cold, and spicy food. Too much caffeine and alcohol can aggravate problems causing irregular periods, so reduce your consumption. It's also a good idea to exercise more and reduce your stress levels. Herb formulations for irregular periods include ingredients like angelica root, white peony root, safflower, and Chinese foxglove.

Cupping for female infertility

Many Traditional Chinese Medicine therapists use cupping to help with infertility, which is caused by any number of factors, including hormonal issues, abdominal disease, problems with the fallopian tubes, stress, and so on. In Traditional Chinese Medicine, cupping tackles the root issues through its improvement of blood circulation. The benefits might include inducing ovulation, removing blockages in the fallopian tubes, balancing issues with thyroid, and so on.

The points on the front of the body are below the belly-button. Look at the first section of your thumb, and remember the length. The first point is about four thumb-lengths below the belly-button, and the second point is slightly lower than that. The other points are on either side of the first pressure point. For the back, two points are located just below the neck. The other three are on the lower back, just above the rear end. They're mirroring the points in the front of the body.

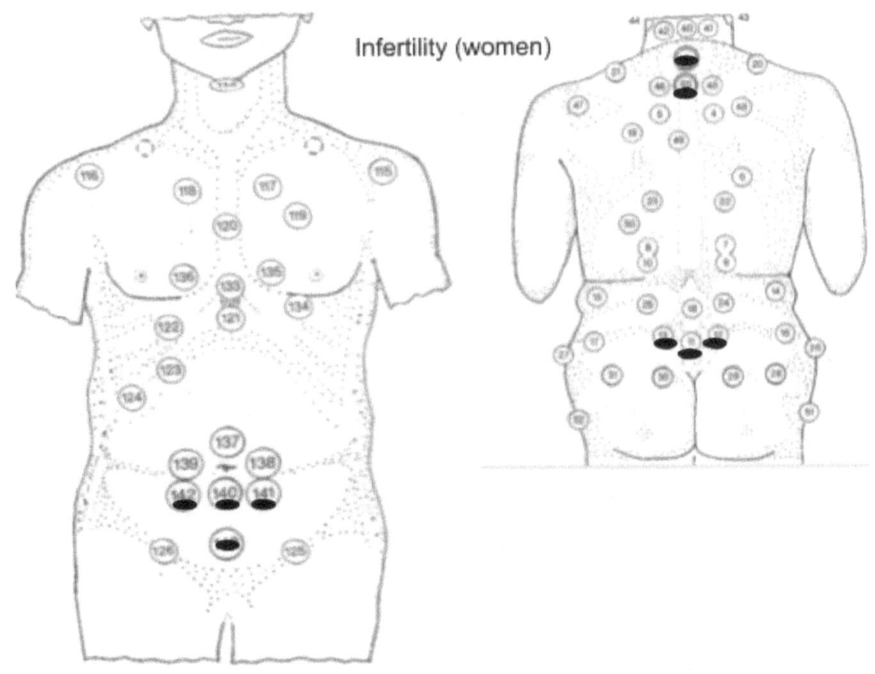

Other treatments for female infertility

Cupping does not "cure" female infertility, because the causes are so varied. It can help remove blockages and stress, but it doesn't assure a pregnancy. Certain foods can also be helpful, like ginger tea and brown-sugar tea. Other foods that can increase libido and fertility include salmon, berries, figs, seaweed, and maca. Avoid mutton, roast beef, and coffee.

Male diseases

Within the umbrella of "male diseases," there's premature ejaculation, male infertility, impotence, and prostatitis. Cupping can be performed all over the body, especially the front and back of the body, the legs, and the bottom of the feet. Let's start by exploring premature ejaculation. Therapists will switch up cupping based on what they believe is causing the problem.

Premature ejaculation

If the therapist believes premature ejaculation is being caused by a kidney deficiency, they will perform vacuum cupping on certain points of the back, front, and foot. The first point on the back is on the lower lumbar, just a smidge to the left of the spine. The other point on the back is below the second cervical vertebrae, in a little cavity you can see marked on the chart. Cupping is performed for 10-15 minutes, followed by moxibustion for 3-5 minutes. On the front of the body, a cup is placed below the navel. There's also a point on the bottom of the foot therapists will cup. They'll massage the point first to warm it up before performing cupping for 10-15 minutes and then moxibustion.

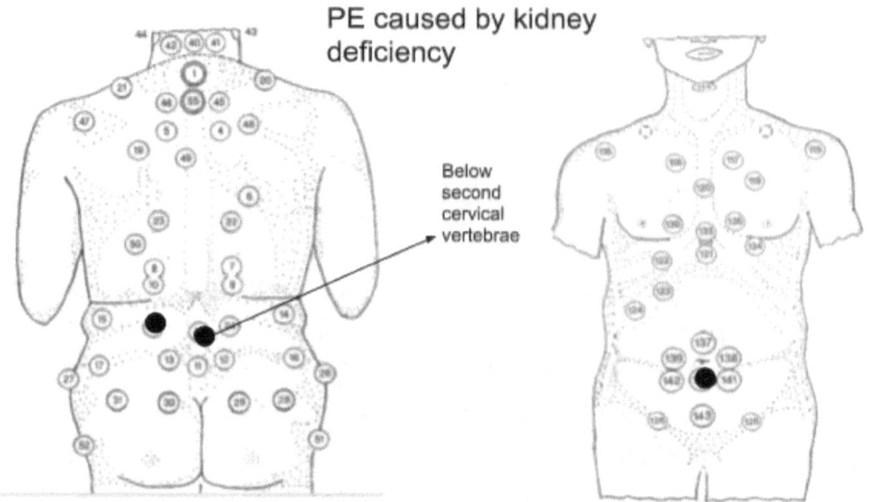

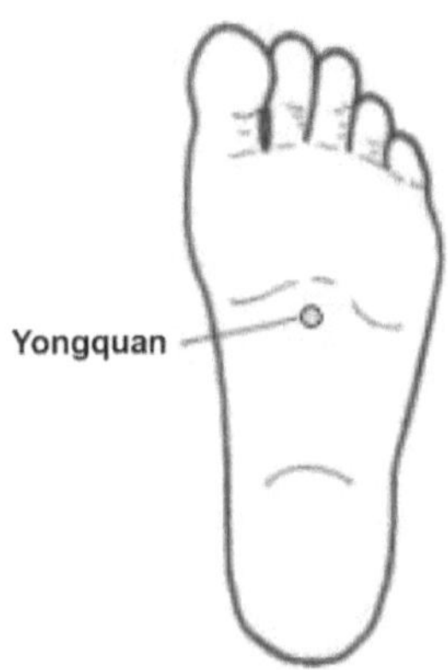

Traditional Chinese Medicine also teaches that premature ejaculation can be caused by "damp heat." This condition causes limb heaviness, skin puffiness, and water retention. It usually arises during the warm summer months. Cupping for damp heat will be performed on the leg, feet, and front. Unlike with premature ejaculation caused by kidney deficiency, therapists probably won't perform moxibustion after a 10-15 minute treatment of stationary suction.

Damp heat

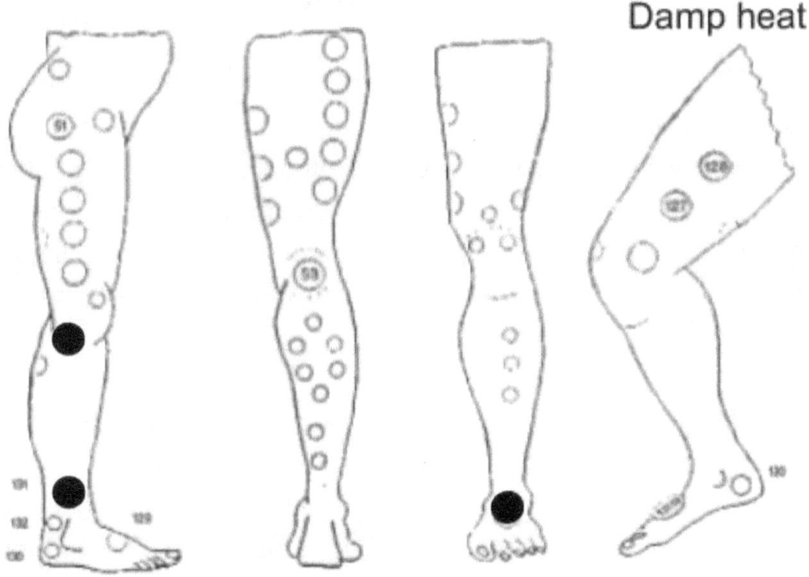

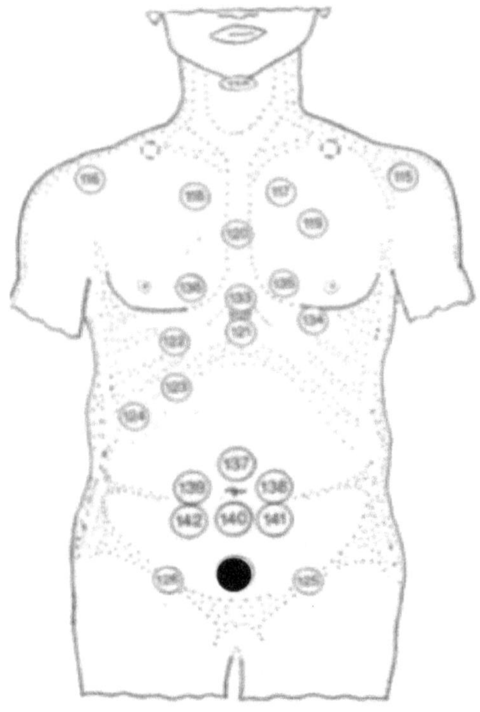

Male infertility

When a couple can't conceive, 35-40% of the time it's because of a health problem in the man. An irregular dilation of veins in the testes can cause improper blood drainage, which heats the area and reduces sperm count. Urinary tract infections and prostatitis can also cause low sperm count. Smoking, chemical exposure, diabetes, hypertension, and problems with the immune system all play a role in infertility.

There are cupping points that can be targeted to help boost male fertility. For the points on the back, moving cupping is applied, with the therapist pushing and pulling on the point. Vacuum cupping can be used afterwards for 10-15 minutes, followed by moxibustion. For the front of the body, there's no massage cupping. Suction is applied, and then moxibustion. For the points on the leg and ankle, the therapist will knead the area to warm it up, suction for 10-15 minutes, and then perform moxibustion.

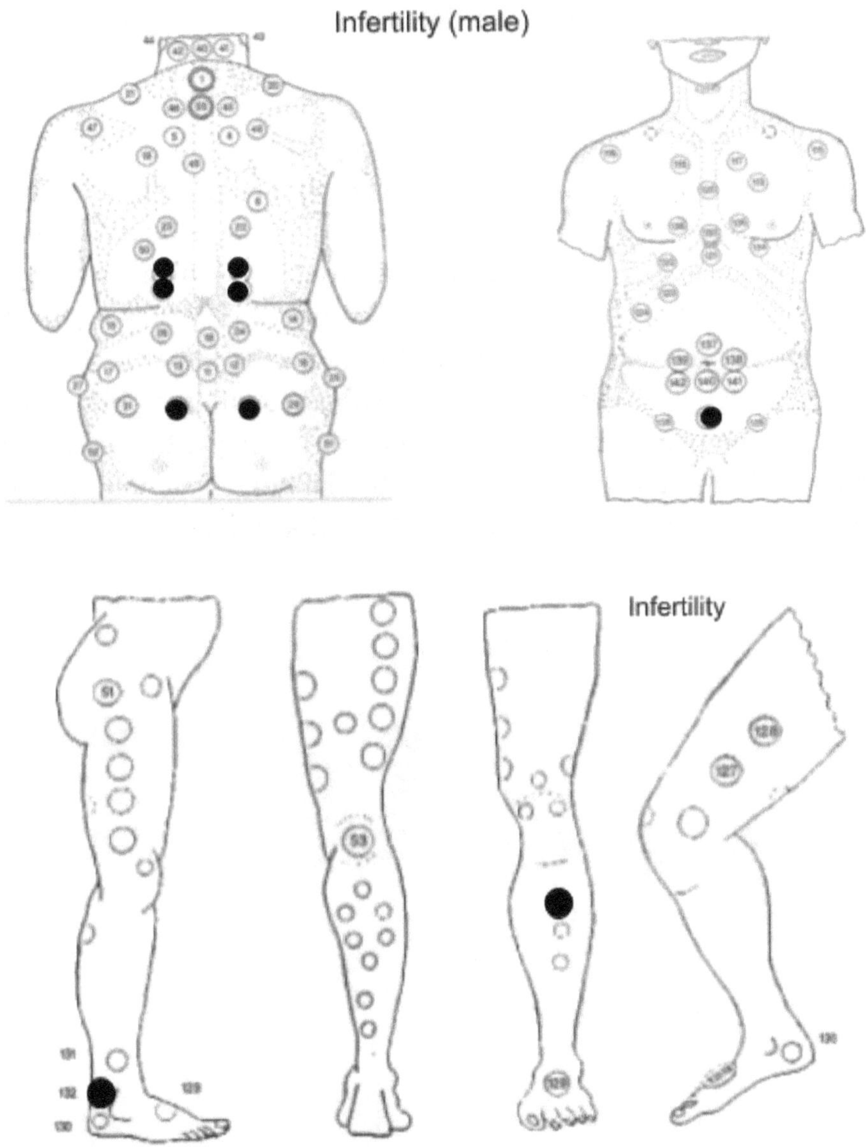

Impotence

Impotence (also known as erectile dysfunction) occurs when a man is unable to achieve an erection or produces a weak erection. Any number of health problems can cause erectile dysfunction, including heart disease, obesity, diabetes, or a sleep disorder. Psychological factors like stress and depression are also common.

Cupping on the back, front, legs, and feet can help remove toxins that might play a role in the condition. The point on the back is found below the second cervical vertebrae, about a hand's width above the buttocks. The point on the front of the body is a few inches below the belly-button. A therapist will cup for 10-15 minutes and then perform moxibustion. The other point is right on the buttocks itself, but there is no moxibustion after cupping. The point on the bottom of the foot should be massaged first and then cupped. The points on the legs and by the ankles are cupped for 10-15 minutes, and then warmed with moxibustion.

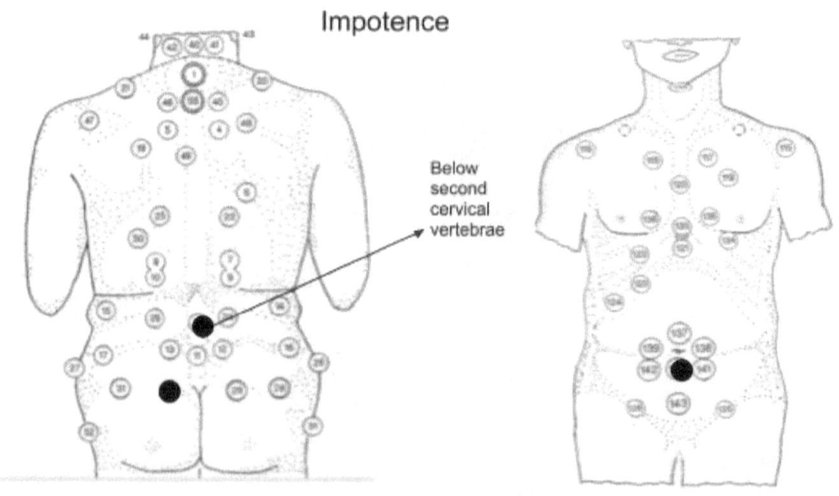

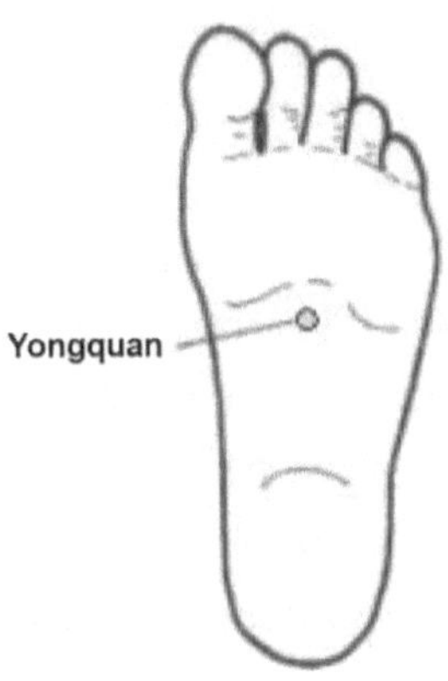

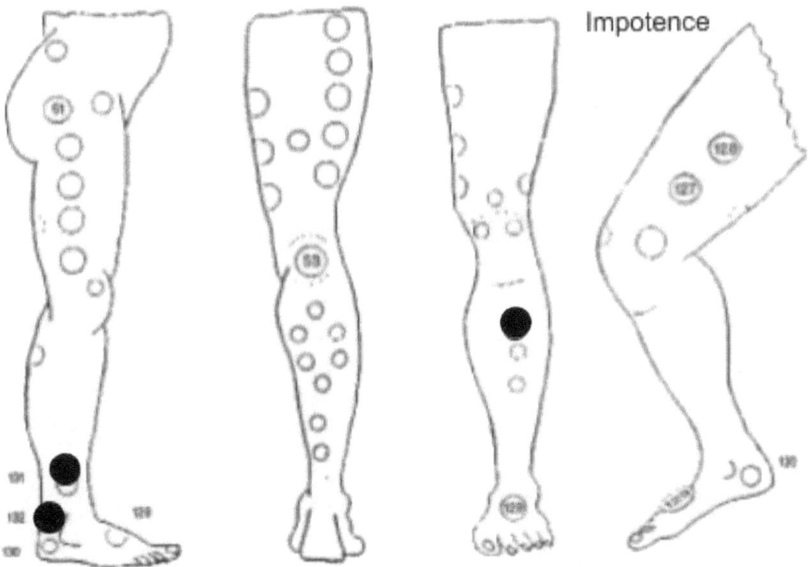

Prostatitis

If a man feels pain while urinating as well as lower waist pain, a lowered desire for sex, and pain during ejaculation, he probably suffers from prostatitis. It's often difficult to pin down the cause, but bacterial infection is commonly-cited. Nerve damage in the lower urinary tract can also cause prostatitis.

For treatment, therapists will perform two sessions of cupping - one group a day. The first group focuses on the back, the front, and the legs. For the points on the back, massage thoroughly back and forth, and then apply suction for 10-15 minutes. On the front, you'll cup for 10-15 minutes below the navel, and on the leg, the therapist will cup on the outer edge of the shin. Moxibustion is often performed afterwards.

For the next day, the therapist will cup on the legs. One is found on the inner edge of the shinbone, with three by the ankle and one a few inches above those. Follow cupping with moxibustion for 3-5 minutes.

1st group Prostatitis

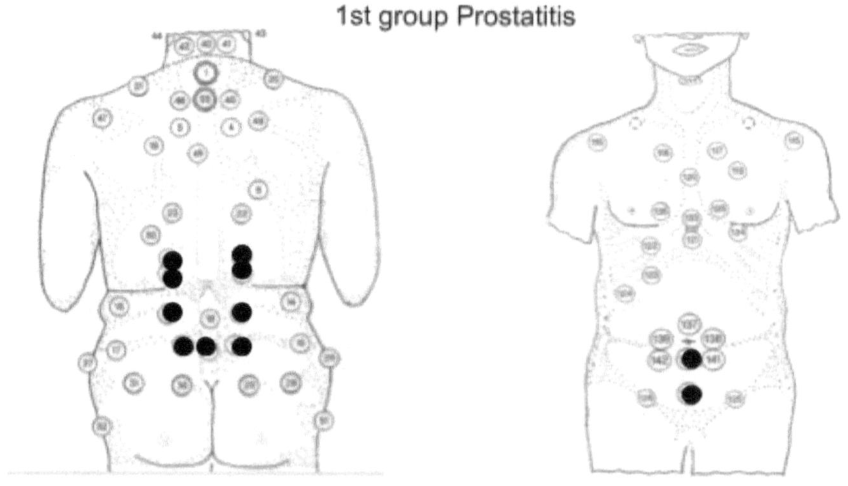

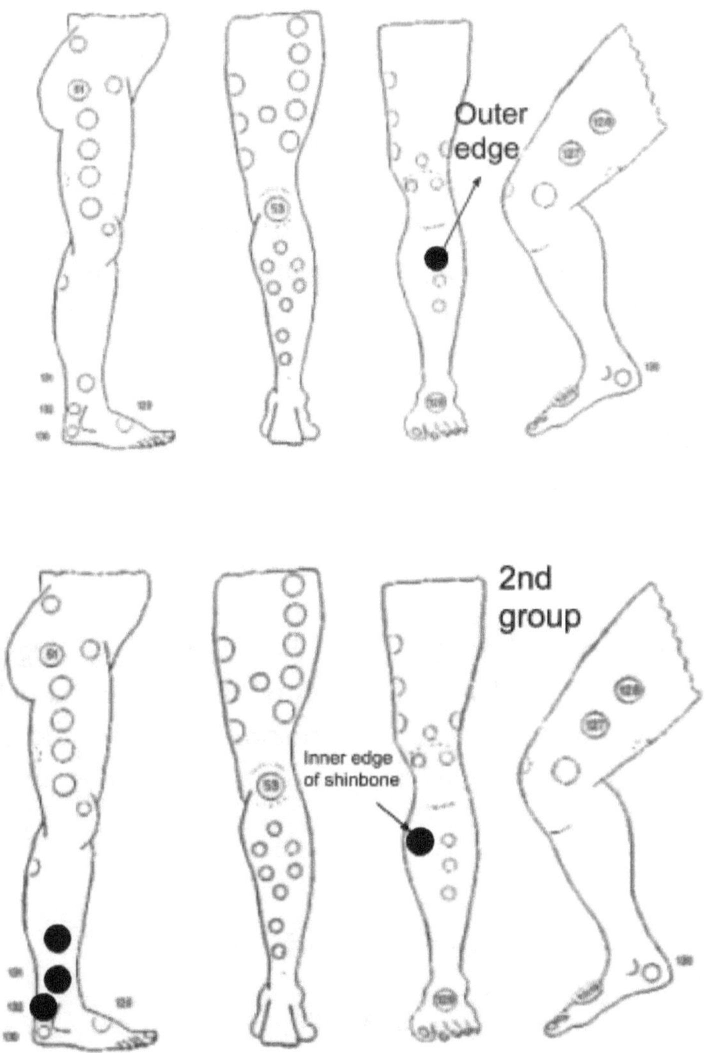

Other treatments for male diseases

Premature ejaculation can be treated by improved emotional regulation. For example, the man should reduce his stress levels and relax during sex. He can also refrain from masturbation and exercise more, which is helpful for reducing stress.

Acupuncture is a common treatment for male infertility, alone or in conjunction with cupping. In terms of what a patient can do on their own, avoiding hot baths and hot tubs can help, as well as not having a laptop right on the lap or wearing tight underwear. If the patient smokes, they should quit. Herbs boost fertility, especially ginseng, saw palmetto, and astragalus. Eat whole foods rich in zinc, vitamin B12, and vitamin E. These improve sperm mobility and production.

Impotence is also very psychological, so treatment will include more relaxing, less stress, and more exercise. The man can also eat more aphrodisiac food and avoid excessive alcohol consumption, soy products, sugar, and junk food.

One's risk of prostatitis can be lowered by engaging in a healthy sex life and always urinating when needed. It's unhealthy to wait. You should also avoid drinking too much alcohol and spicy food. Healthy foods include kelp, red beans, citrus, and berries.

Treating colds and congestion

In Traditional Chinese Medicine, fevers, colds, and chills all begin with an invasion of "wind." The wind is either cold or hot; they're known as "wind-cold" and "wind-heat." This refers to the first stages of a sickness where you flip between feeling too cold or too hot. Your body is fighting off the symptoms, and cupping can help. By pulling the "winds" to the surface through cupping, you can clear them away. Cupping also strengthens the respiratory system, better preparing it to handle the next wave of congestion-causing toxins that comes through town.

To begin, the therapist will apply oil to the upper back. They might use an essential oil like eucalyptus or a blend with peppermint and lavender. The cup is then applied on the back, and glided around in an up-and-down motion on both sides of the spine. Circulator motions might also be used. The standard therapy lasts 10 minutes or longer, depending on how congested you are. The therapist may also perform the same treatment on your chest. Other points for cold symptoms (sore throat, sinuses) are labeled in the graphs on the next page.

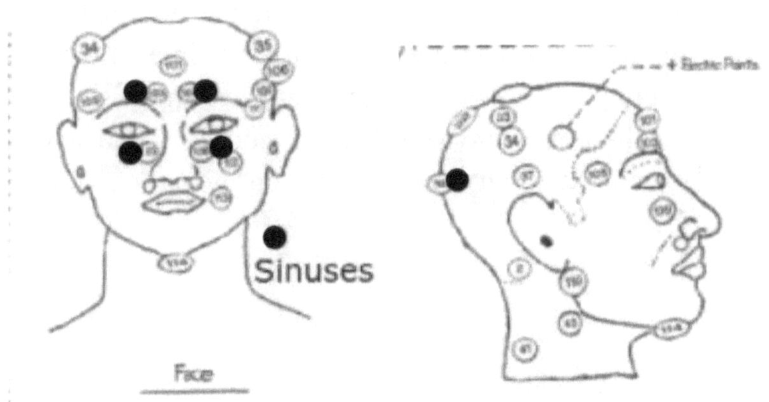

Other treatments for colds + congestion

Acupuncture is a very common treatment for colds and congestion. In Traditional Chinese Medicine, the goal is to "push out" the germs, and not kill them. That means antibiotics are typically not used. For diet, warm and soothing food like miso soup and ginger tea is recommended if you have a headache and mild chills. If you feel hot, however, warming food isn't good. Yin Qiao San is a popular cooling herb formula. Stay hydrated and get lots of quality rest.

Vomiting and nausea

A lot of factors can cause vomiting and nausea, including pregnancy, headaches, illness, the environment, and more. We cover many of the underlying causes in this book, but what do you do to treat the symptom? One of the most effective points for treating vomiting and nausea is on the inner forearm between the two tendons. It's called P6 or "Nei Guan," in Chinese. It's been proven in scientific studies to reduce the nausea and vomiting during pregnancy and following surgeries.

Cupping should be performed on the dominant hand for just 3-5 minutes. You can cup as often as 3 times a day. There's also a pressure point below the knee that can help. It's on the outer edge of the shinbone, and you'll know you've found it when the muscle flexes under your finger when you move your foot up and down.

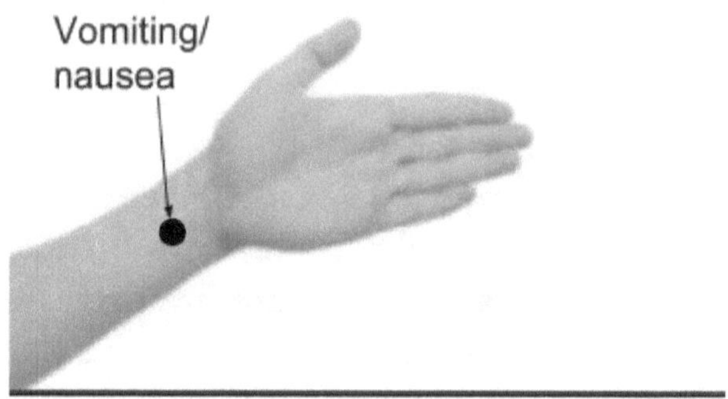

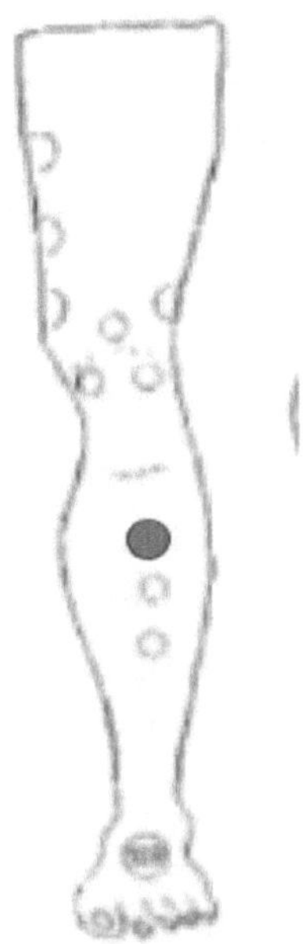

Other treatments for vomiting/nausea

The correct herbs and diet are essential for relieving nausea and recovering from vomiting. Chamomile and ginger tea are both effective, especially for morning sickness. Tarragon and peppermint teas are also popular. Herb formulations will include ginger, cardamom, licorice, and Chinese basil. For your diet, you should avoid heavy and rich foods after vomiting, and rely on clear liquids. Avoid preservatives and foods with additives. Since vomiting and nausea are often caused by indigestion, eat foods that help with the digestive system, including pineapples, papayas, yams, potatoes, and brown rice. Avoid hard-to-digest food like dairy. Stay hydrated.

Treating lung/breathing problems

Part of your cold might include a cough and other breathing issues. Other separate lung problems include asthma and bronchitis. These are caused by a buildup of phlegm in the lungs.

Excessive phlegm is a result of viral or bacterial infections, inhaled irritants, or allergies. Other causes include pregnancy and smoking. Your lymphatic system and the body's ability to drain fluids properly gets disrupted, so that's what cupping targets.

The therapist will apply oil to the back in line with the lungs. Essential oils like wintergreen, peppermint, and eucalyptus encourage deep, healthy breathing. The cups are placed on the body with a light or medium suction, and then left for 10 minutes or so. The therapist might also apply massage cupping around this area. Massage cupping can also be done beginning on either side of the spine and slid out toward the armpit, all the way down the back. Circulator motions are good, and a treatment of 10 minutes helps drain the lymphatic system.

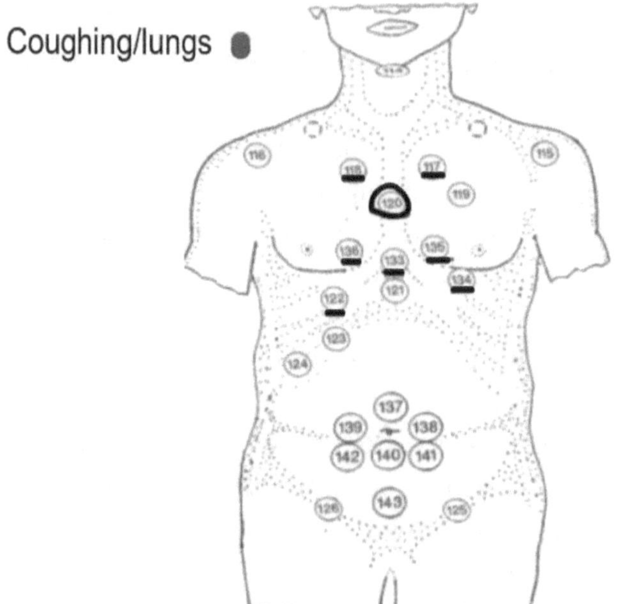

Other treatments for lung/breathing problems

For a cough, it's a good idea to increase your exercise a bit to build up your body's strength and resistance to disease. Getting outside time is especially beneficial, provided the air isn't polluted. As you work out, you should be prepared to remove or put on clothing if you feel too hot or cold.

For treating asthma, you should avoid pets, allergens, and dampness, as this causes mold to grow. Make sure your home is free from mold and dust. During the spring, you need to keep your windows and doors closed. For food, avoid overly-spicy and greasy food like seafood, peppers, onions, and garlic.

If you're suffering from bronchitis, avoid substances that irritate your lungs. Make sure the air inside your home is clean and circulating. Clean dust from your home, too, but be careful of harsh chemical cleaners. If you smoke, you need to quit. Increasing your amount of exercise can also be helpful in building up lung strength.

Cupping for high cholesterol/hypertension

High cholesterol is linked to high blood pressure (hypertension), and increases a person's risk for heart attack or stroke because it limits blood flow. Over time, the blood thickens and gets heavier. Cholesterol coats the walls of the arteries, narrowing them and thickening the cells, so the heart has to work harder. High blood pressure can be traced back to obesity, smoking, chronic heart disease, genetics, stress, and poor nutrition.

Cupping can help move out the stagnant blood, replacing it with healthy blood. Cupping might also help regulate the sodium in your body, which causes high cholesterol. Studies connecting cupping and health benefits focus on wet cupping, and show that it may prevent clogged arteries, improve blood circulation, and balance blood iron levels.

There are quite a few pressure points that treat high cholesterol and hypertension, and they're actually on the back. As you can see in the chart, many of them are located on the middle and lower back. A therapist might use both regular dry cupping or massage cupping. While cupping can be beneficial for heart health, it should not be done on anyone with a pacemaker.

For cupping on the lower back with points, the therapist will massage the points up and down, and then apply suction for 10-15 minutes. Stationary cupping is applied higher up on the neck and below the neck. A therapist might apply cupping on the back one day, and then while those marks fade, they perform another session on the legs and feet. The area is warmed first with a finger massage, and then cupped for 10-15 minutes. Some websites say those with heart disease shouldn't be treated at all with cupping, so to be safe, consult a doctor first, and only have it performed by a professional.

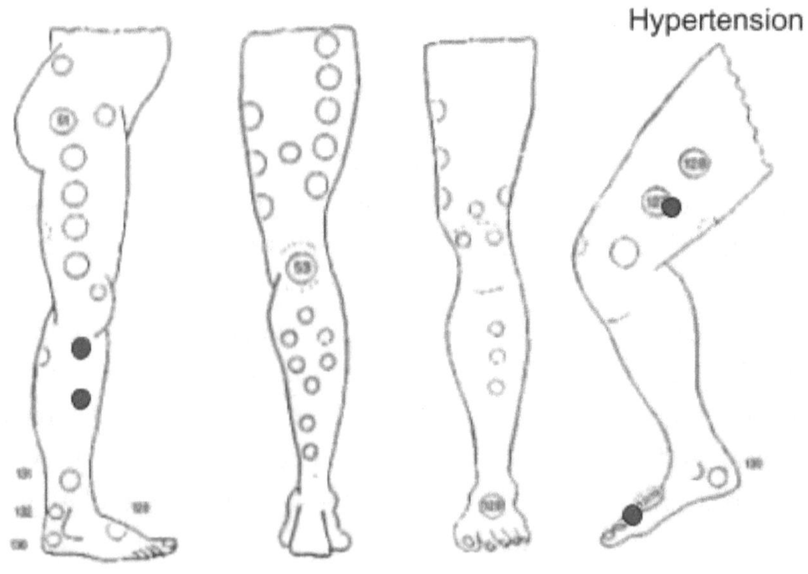

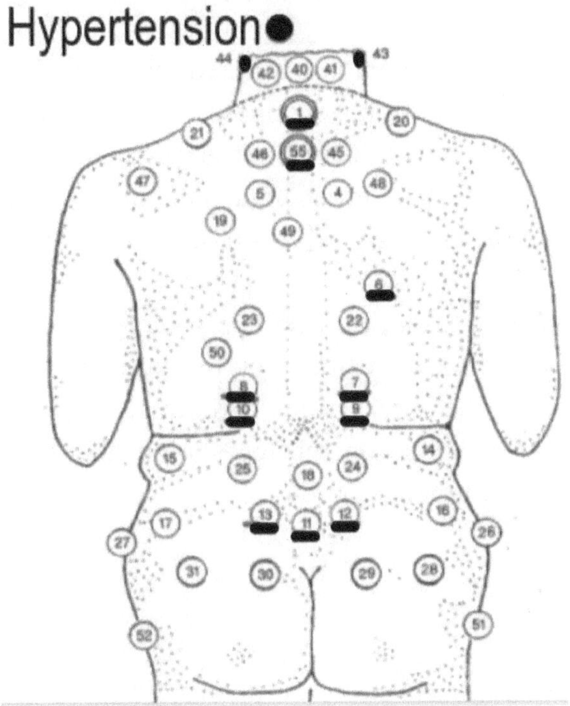

Other treatments for hypertension

Treating high blood pressure and hypertension requires a balance of rest, exercise, and positive emotions. You should avoid spicy food, smoking, and too much alcohol. While going through a cupping treatment, it's safe to be on medication (antihypertensive meds), but you should gradually reduce it. Herbs like celery seed, garlic, flaxseed, and hibiscus tea can lower blood pressure.

Anemia

Those with anemia have a red blood cell deficiency. It causes fatigue, pale skin, dizziness, and palpitations. Causes include iron deficiency, kidney disease, pregnancy, poor nutrition, or chronic illness. Sickle cell anemia is hereditary and is caused by a problem with the body's production of hemoglobins.

For the points on the back, apply suction for 10-15 minutes, and then perform moxibustion. For the point at the front of the body, massage the area first and then apply suction and moxibustion. The points on the leg should also be massaged by hand first before cupping.

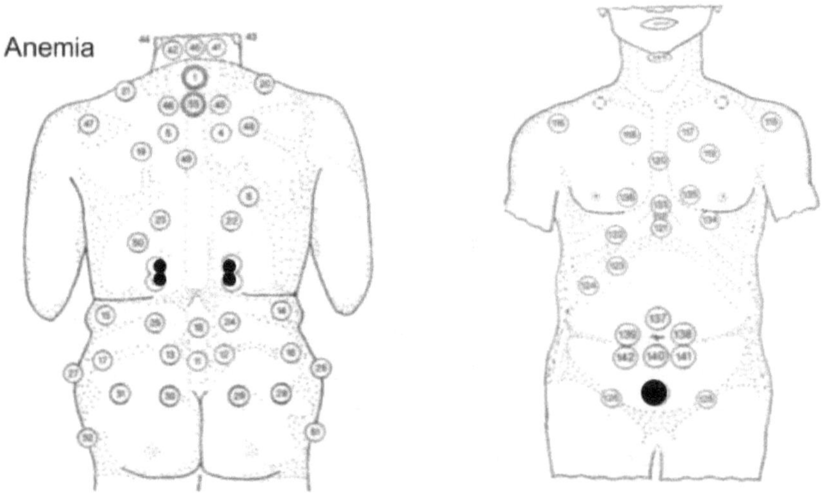

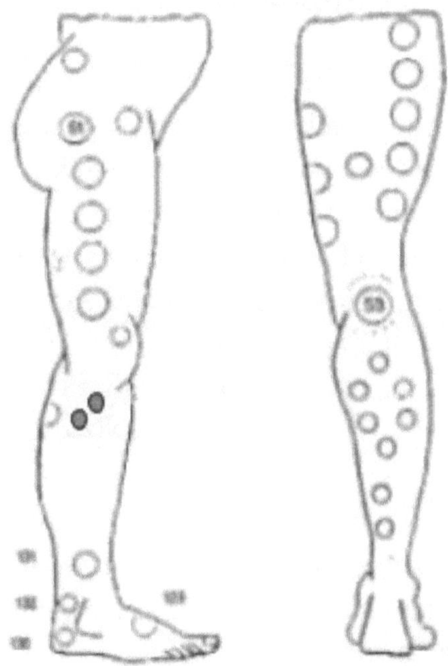

Other treatments for anemia

In Traditional Chinese Medicine, anemia is believed to be caused by stagnant blood or qi, so promoting good circulation is key. Both acupuncture and cupping are usually performed. Ginseng is commonly prescribed, as are dang shen (a root that boosts hemoglobin production) and bu zhong yi wan, a formulation of herbs designed to increase energy and hemoglobins. Patients should eat foods rich in vitamin C, folic acid, zinc, iron, and vitamin B12.

Cupping for diabetes

Much discussion has surrounded diabetes and cupping, and whether or not it's a safe or helpful procedure. Benefits could include more balanced nutrients in the body, specifically glucose, iron, cholesterol, and calcium. Cupping could also improve a patient's movement and flexibility, thanks to cupping's ability to get circulation going. However, diabetics may also face increased risk because of their lowered immunity. Cupping is not recommended for Stage 4 diabetics.

You can see on the chart where the relevant points are for diabetes. Because of the increased risk, diabetics should not try cupping at home. The professional should always be told about the patient's condition, since the patient will need to make sure their blood sugar is at a good level and stays that way through the session.

On the back, the points will be massaged and suctioned. The therapist will massage up and down on the points, which are on the upper back and lower back. They should also be suctioned for 10-15 minutes afterwards. For the legs, knead the points with your thumb first to warm up the area, then vacuum-cup for 10 minutes or so. Find the little hollow behind the ankle bone, by the Achilles tendon. The other points are higher up on the leg at the bottom of the shin, and then below the knee on the inner edge of the shin bone.

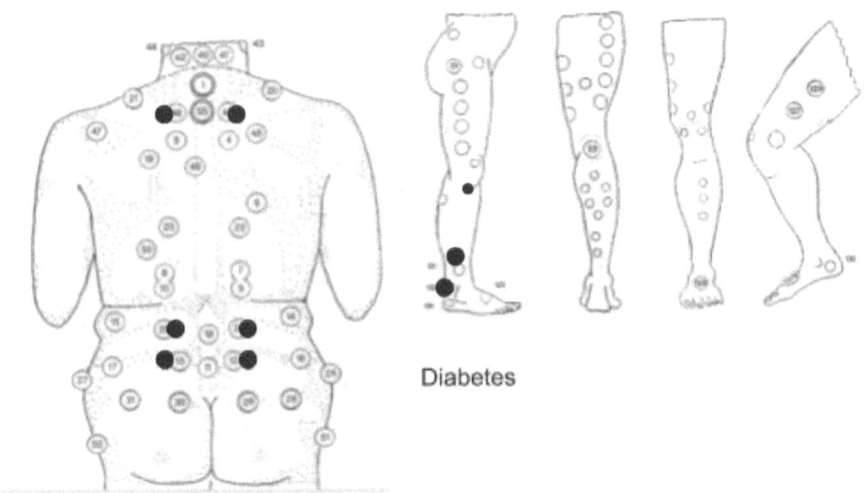

Diabetes

Other treatments for diabetes

Paying attention to one's diet and exercise is important for treating diabetes. Patients should continue to take the proper medication to control blood sugar. In terms of herbs, Korean ginseng and balsam pear are commonly used. Acupuncture is also a popular treatment.

Treating foot pain

Everyone from athletes to servers in the food industry feel foot pain. It can be debilitating and cause pain all over the body. Some also suffer from what's known as "plantar fasciitis," a deep, aching pain in the arch of the foot and bottom of the heel. The foot contains deep muscles that connect to the legs and hips, so healing foot pain can affect your whole body. Benefits of foot cupping include better blood circulation, relief from pain, and relief from stiff muscles.

For cupping on the feet, therapists stick to the fleshiest parts. The points are between and beside bony areas, tendons, and ligaments. You never cup on a bone or over an artery. Using small cups, therapists glide around oiled fleshy areas on the bottom of the foot with a weak or medium suction, including the heel. Therapists can also cup on the top of the foot and around the ankles and calf.

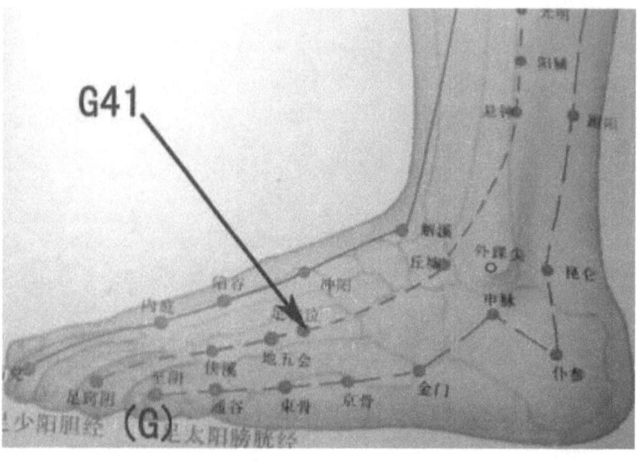

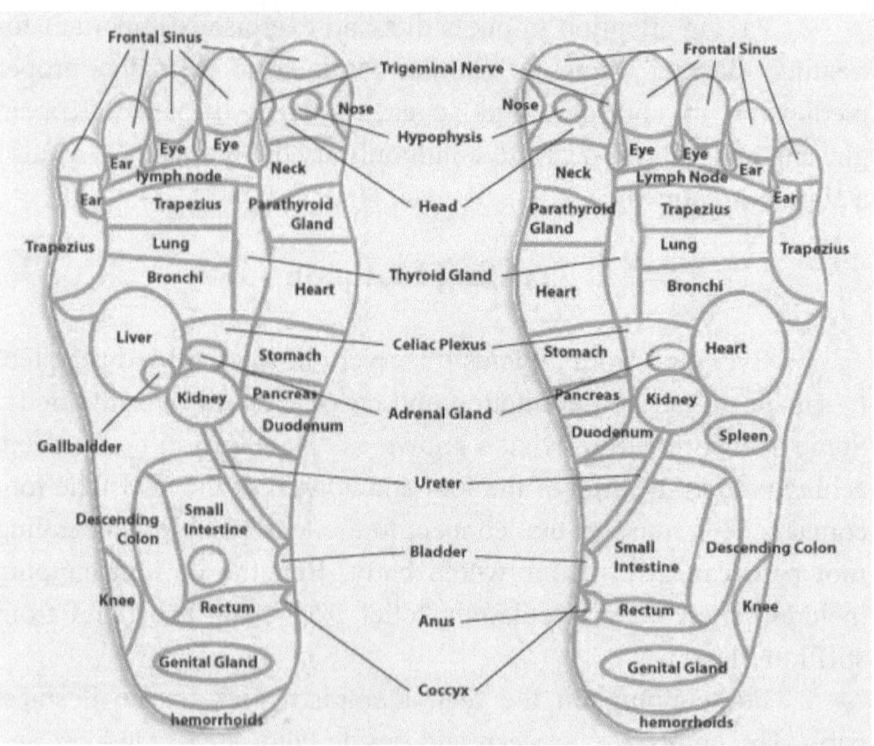

As you can see in the above images, there are a lot of pressure points in the feet. They correspond to other parts of the body like organs and functions, but to keep things simple, focus on the points on or close to the area of pain on your foot. You should never feel sharp pain when cupping on the foot. You will see points in the foot referenced for other conditions.

Other treatments for foot pain

Regular massage is very effective at treating foot pain, as is acupuncture. In Traditional Chinese Medicine, plantar fasciitis is caused by problems with the kidney and liver. Therapists will massage, cup, and perform acupuncture on the parts of the food that correspond to those organs. Soaking your feet in a warm bath with epsom salt is a common remedy for foot pain. Some people even steep their feet in tea, either peppermint or chamomile. To prevent foot pain, you can also wear thicker, shock-absorbing shoe soles, which is a good option for those whose pain is caused by long hours on their feet.

Leg cramps/soreness in leg and ankle

Leg cramps occur when you work out, stand a lot, or if you aren't getting enough calcium and potassium. Leg cramps can also occur at night if you aren't warm enough. There are three points on each leg that can be massaged and cupped. The first point can be found on the outer side of the shin. The second is right in the crease at the back of the knee, where the arrow is pointing. The last is at the back of the lower leg between the two big muscles. The therapist should massage the points with their thumb first for 2-3 minutes, until the point actually feels sore, like it's beginning to swell. Apply suction for 5-10 minutes.

The image is specific to the right leg, but the points mirror each other on the left. For muscle soreness in the leg and ankle, massage the back of the knee for a few minutes, then apply suction for 5-10 minutes. That point (called "Weizhong" in Traditional Chinese Medicine) connects to the leg, ankle, hip, and can treat a range of conditions.

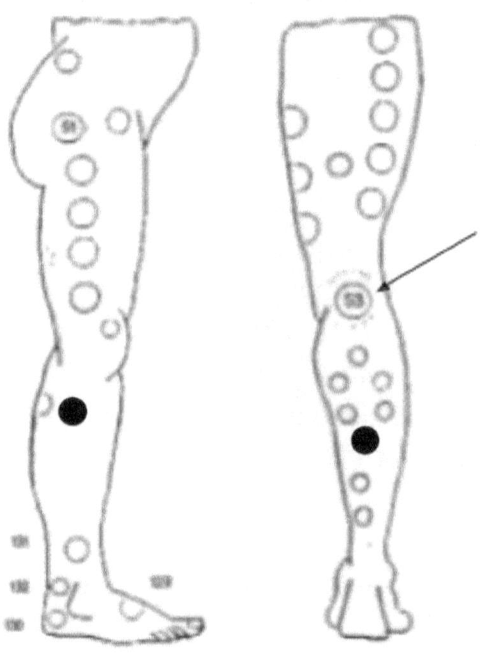

Other treatments for cramps and soreness

Along with cupping, you can adopt healthy habits to improve leg cramps and muscle soreness. If cramps are coming on because of exercise, be sure to warm up the muscles before a workout, and slow down. Consume more calcium by drinking milk and other high-calcium foods. Proper hydration is also essential. For those who feel like their muscles are always sore, rest by avoiding high-intensity exercise for a while. If your leg cramps come at night, it could be caused by cold, so be sure to stay warm. Stretching before bed can help, too.

Varicosity

Varicosity is characterized by swelling, fatigue, aching, and enlarged veins, especially in the legs and feet. These are called "varicose veins," and appear more often in women than men. Causes include obesity, aging, leg injury, pregnancy, and standing for too long. It's also hereditary.

Cupping points for varicosity are found on the middle back, foot, and above the knee. For the points on the back, cupping is performed on either side of the spine for 10-15 minutes, followed by moxibustion. On the foot, the therapists massages the area with their thumb first, and then cups for 10-15 minutes. The point above the knee, on the inner side, is also massaged and then cupped.

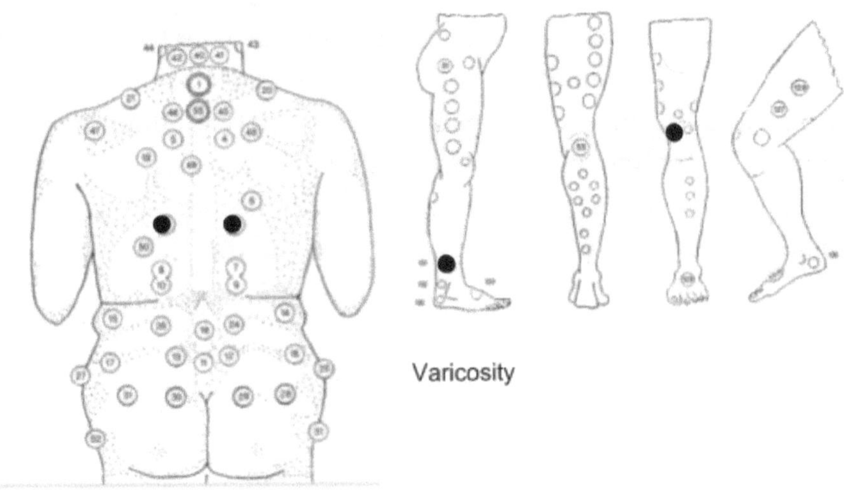

Varicosity

Other treatments for varicosity

If a patient has varicosity, they should avoid standing for long periods of time and get plenty of rest. According to Traditional Chinese Medicine, varicose veins are caused by low qi in the spleen, since it is the spleen's job to maintain veins. A therapist might also perform acupuncture to raise the spleen's qi. In terms of herbs and food, horse chestnut is effective, while foods rich in antioxidants can strengthen the affected veins.

Hemorrhoids

Hemorrhoids are swollen, inflamed veins in the anus and rectum. They're basically varicose veins. They often bleed and are quite painful. Causes include pregnancy, obesity, chronic diarrhea, chronic constipation, and straining too hard to make a bowel movement. Women are more likely to suffer from them when they're pregnant, and one's risk goes up with age.

For a cupping treatment, therapists focus on the back and one point on the leg. For the points on the upper back, apply suction for 10-15 minutes. For the ones on the lower back, move the cup around until the skin becomes red. Apply suction for 10-15 minutes. The points on the buttocks should also be massaged with the cup until the skin reddens, and then suctioned for 10-15 minutes. Apply suction to the leg for 10-15 minutes.

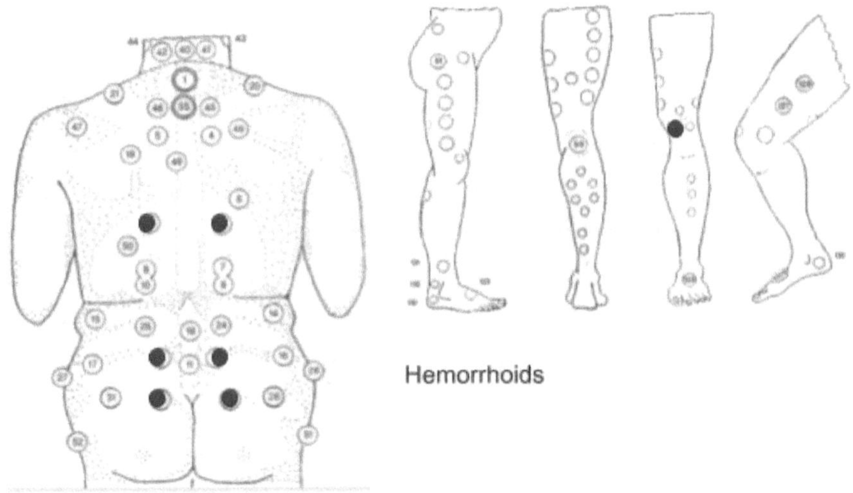

Hemorrhoids

Other treatments for hemorrhoids

To prevent hemorrhoids, avoid spicy food. Instead, eat foods like vegetables, bananas, and other high-fiber foods. Always go to the bathroom when you need to, but don't strain. Foods like prunes, flaxseed, green beans, rice, and spinach can relieve constipation.

To treat hemorrhoids, a short 15-minute bath can relieve pain and shrink the veins. Afterwards, carefully dry the area. Ointments made with aloe vera can also help. In Traditional Chinese Medicine, ginkgo biloba and horse chestnut as a supplement are often prescribed.

Treating hand pain

Carpal tunnel syndrome is a tingling pain located in your hand and wrist. It can also be felt in the thumb, index finger, middle finger, and ring finger. The little finger is usually spared because it's controlled by a different nerve. CTS is often triggered by working on a computer a lot. In a study, researchers cupped patients with carpal tunnel syndrome for 5-10 minutes in the shoulder muscle that affects the aggravated nerve. They treated a second group for 15 minutes with a heating pad. The cupping group improved better, with a 60% reduction of symptoms. You can see pressure points for CTS in the image below:

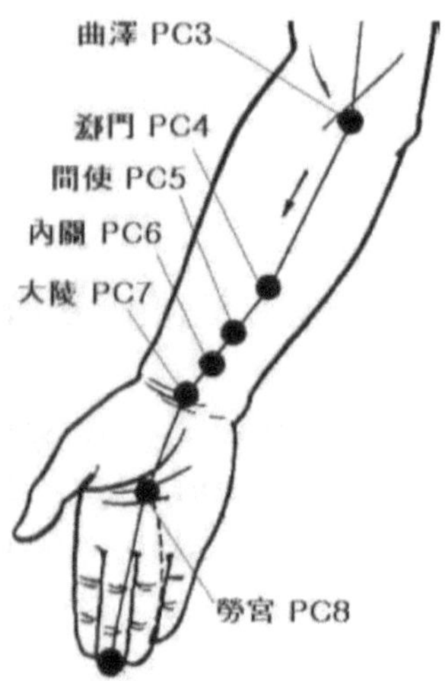

While we're talking about hands, it's worth mentioning how the hands (like the feet) are a hotbed of pressure points that affect the whole body. As you can see in the graph below, the hands are mirrors of each other and match up with the feet.

Hand Reflexology Chart

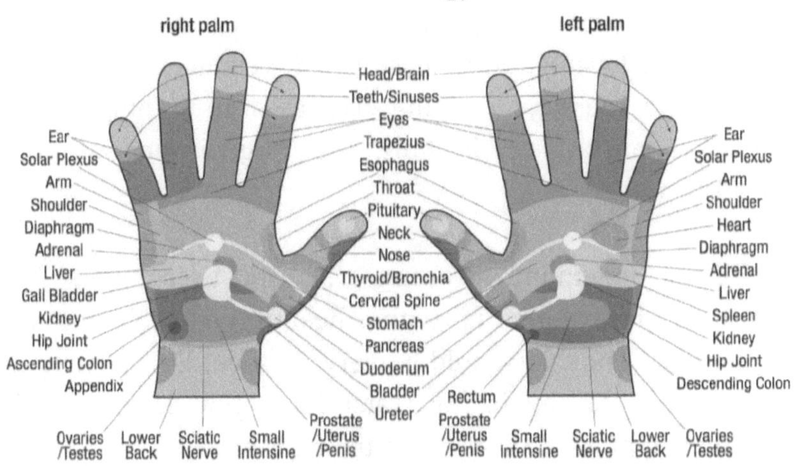

Other treatments for hand pain

Massage and acupuncture complement cupping when it comes to hand pain. Hand exercises can also help loosen and stretch the hand muscles, while soaking your hands in hot water for 10-15 minutes soothes sore joints and improves circulation. Research has also shown that extract from the Tripterygium wilfordii plant (the thunder god vine) is very effective at treating inflammation, swelling, and joint pain. Some therapists will also recommend splinting the wrist in a straight position (especially for carpal tunnel), which reduces pressure on the nerve.

Cupping for physical therapy/sport injuries

Athletes use cupping to stretch their muscles, work out tension, and recover from injuries. Dr. Bahram Jam describes what he calls "Tissue Distraction Release w/ Movement," which sounds essentially like massage cupping. He uses it to help promote healing after an athlete is hurt. He targets the soft tissue specifically.

Before beginning cupping, the soft-tissue area being cupped should be warmed up with a heating pad or 5 minutes of cardio exercise. The cup should be very flexible; Dr. Jam suggests rinsing the silicone cup in hot water for a few seconds. Oil or cream is then applied to the area, so the cups glide easily.

Certain areas will cause more discomfort than others. The gluteal and calf muscles are especially sensitive. There are three movements: longitudinal, cross-fiber, and circular. Longitudinal means that the cup moves up and down the area, relaxing tension and loosening muscles. Cross-fiber can cause more discomfort. This is because the massage is working to break down knots and lesions caused by injuries like sprains, breaks, or tears. The cup should move on the skin back and forth in a straight line, and then up and down. You should *not* attempt cross-fiber massage on areas that are swollen, red, or recently-hurt. Always start cupping cautiously, and monitor how the patient feels.

In one case treating a strain injury, therapist Brandi Ross treated an athlete with a strain in his calf. When Dr. Ross began using a cup over the area, she could literally hear the sound of grit. This sound was caused by adhesions, which is scar tissue binding tissue that doesn't normally go together. After just one treatment, the athlete reported back with more flexibility and no pain, and so continued with the cupping.

The last cupping movement is circular, which is performed by making circles with the cup to ensure that all the tissue in the affected area gets covered. Remove the cup and have the patient rest during clean-up. If the patient reports back and says they feel worse, don't repeat the treatment. If the patient feels fine, the therapist will usually strengthen the suction and massage for a bit longer than before. Like with regular physical therapy, the strength of the treatment increases as the patient is able to handle more. The image shows common injury areas in the leg therapists will encounter:

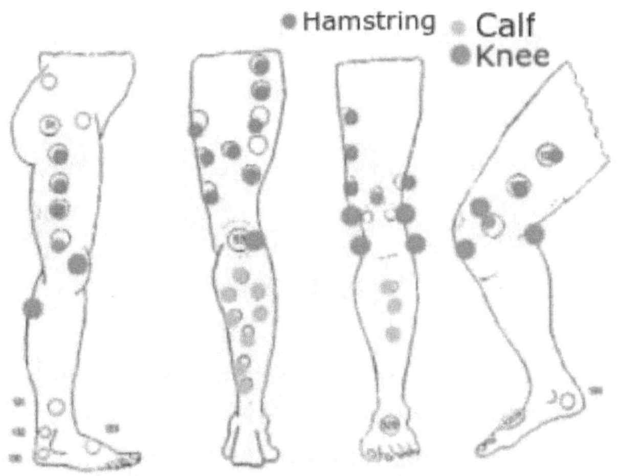

Shoulder + neck soreness

Soreness in the shoulders and neck are common for athletes. It's also common for anyone with stress. There are two places therapists will cup. Between the neck and shoulder on both sides of the body, you'll find an important pressure point. Therapists will rub it for a few minutes to warm it up, and then perform vacuum-cupping for 5-10 minutes.

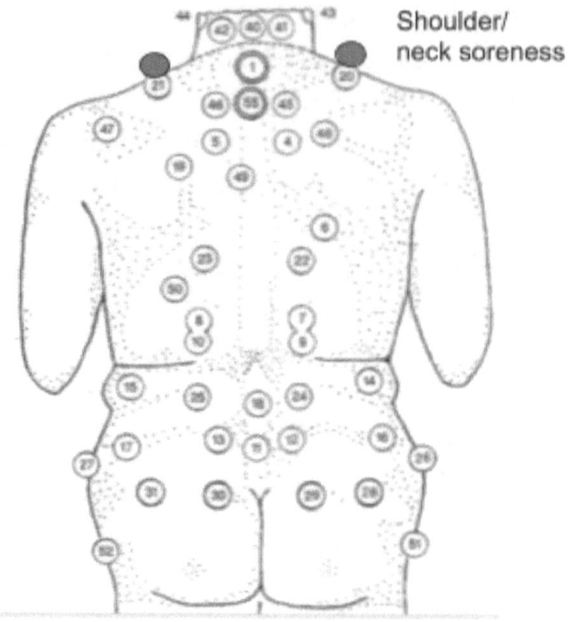

Other treatments for physical therapy and sport injuries

Acupuncture is used in physical therapy and for treating sport injuries because it promotes pain relief and healing. When it comes to other treatments, Traditional Chinese Medicine differs from Western techniques in that it does *not* use ice or compression to reduce inflammation and swelling. Instead, it uses herbs like "Three Yellow Powder," or San Huang San. It's made of three cooling herbs that boost circulation. It's used for sprains, muscle pulls, and strains.

Soaking in alternating hot and cold water is recommended by Traditional Chinese Medicine 1-2 days after acupuncture, massage, and/or cupping. Plasters and poultices are also used. A plaster is a dressing treated with healing herbs. When applied to the injury, it relieves pain and stimulates circulation. Poultices are similar, but they aren't put on a dressing. The herbs are put directly on the body. These are also recommended for arthritis.

For muscle soreness, be sure to stay warm and dry during damp and cold weather, which can aggravate the pain. Careful stretching and exercise is also beneficial, as it prevents muscles from seizing up.

Shoulder pain

Shoulder pain that feels sharp and cutting, like a knife, affects the whole arm and body. If not treated properly, it turns into stiffness and might result in the loss of movement. Keeping the area warm is very important, and therapists will often perform both cupping and acupuncture. There are two point groups therapists focus on - one group one day, and then the other group the next day while the initial marks fade.

The first group focuses on the shoulder area itself. All three points should be massaged by hand first to ensure the points are warm. On the pressure point indicated by the largest dot, the cup should be applied for 15-20 minutes. The therapist will likely then perform moxibustion for just 3-5 minutes. For the smaller point, the pressure point can be found just above the crease where the arm meets the back. The last point in the 1st group mirrors the first point on the shoulder below the collarbone.

For the second group, you actually target the legs. On the back of the leg, the point is between the two muscles of the calf, in the middle of the lower leg. Apply suction for 10-15 minutes. The points on the front of the leg on the shin on the outer side. Apply suction for 10-15 minutes.

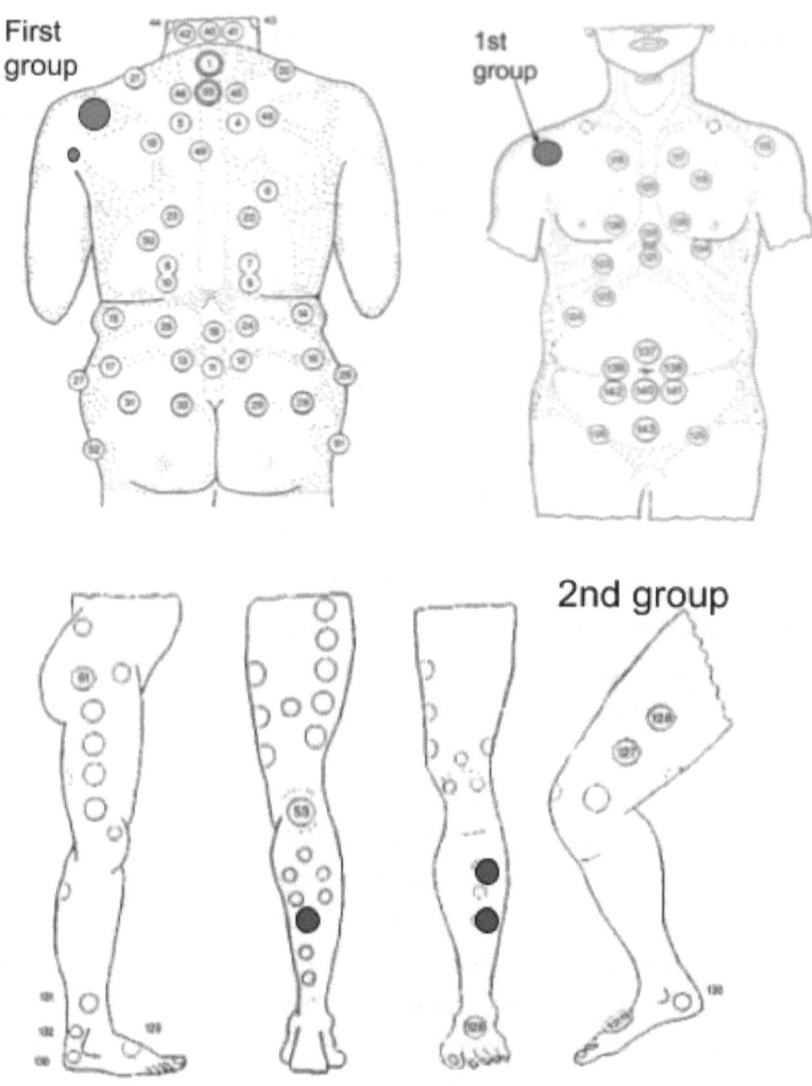

Other treatments for shoulder pain

When you're dealing with shoulder pain, it's very important to keep the area warm. Wear clothes that cover the area and stay warm at night. This encourages good blood circulation, which heals the area. You should also do shoulder joint exercises. Therapists will probably use cupping, massage, and acupuncture. Prescribed herb formulations include white peony, ginger, angelica, and other ingredients meant to drive out dampness and cold.

Rheumatoid arthritis

Arthritic pain involves swelling of the joints in certain areas, especially the hands, wrists, and feet. Causes vary and can include injuries, abnormal metabolism, an infection, an immune system dysfunction, or even just genetics.

For cupping, the therapist will focus on your specific area of pain. After rubbing the painful areas to warm them, they will apply suction. Cupping should not be performed on small joints. A therapist might also perform cupping on a patient's back. For the points on the upper back, you'll apply cups for 15-20 minutes on either side of the spine below shoulders and neck. For the lower back, the points can be found just above the buttocks on both sides of the spine.

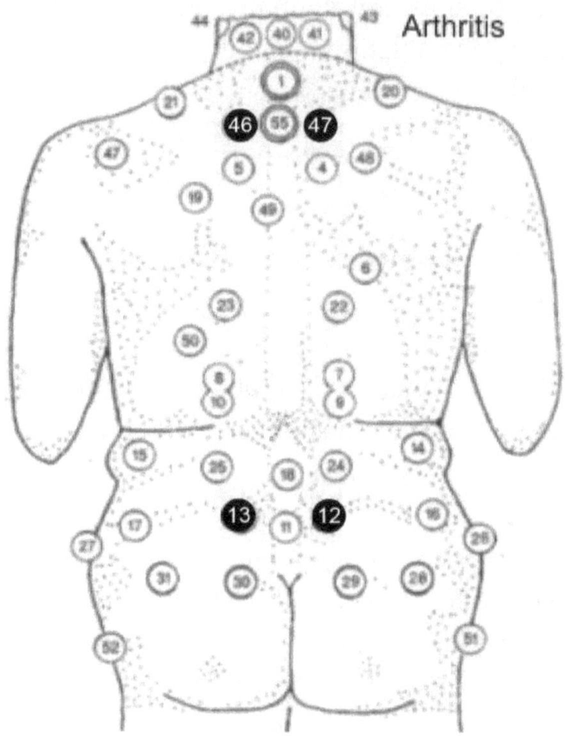

Other treatments for arthritis

When a patient has arthritis, they should be careful about their diet. Avoid dairy, fatty meat, sugar, alcohol, coffee, tea, and foods high in cholesterol. It's good to eat food high in arginine, histidine, and collagen, like eggs, fish, shrimp, beans, potatoes, chicken, and lean beef. If they smoke, they should stop.

In addition to cupping and acupuncture, a therapist might also use plasters and poultices to treat arthritic pain. Various herbs will be used such as ginger extract, licorice, and cinnamon oil.

Gout

Gout is a type of arthritis caused when uric acid crystals buildup in the joints. Normally, uric acid is produced when chemical compounds called "purines" get broken down. The kidneys eliminate the acid through urine, but when the body has too much purine or there's a problem with the kidneys, the buildup occurs. Eating too much of the food which contains purines (red meat, seafood, refined carbs, sugar) can trigger excess. Gout causes severe joint pain, swelling, and redness, especially in the big toe. Attacks of pain often occur in the middle of the night.

Cupping for gout treatment should be performed on the lower lumbar and around the ankles. The cup should be placed on the back for 10-15 minutes, followed by moxibustion to warm the area. For the feet, therapists focus on the ankle and any other affected areas. The points should be massaged first and then cupped for 10-15 minutes.

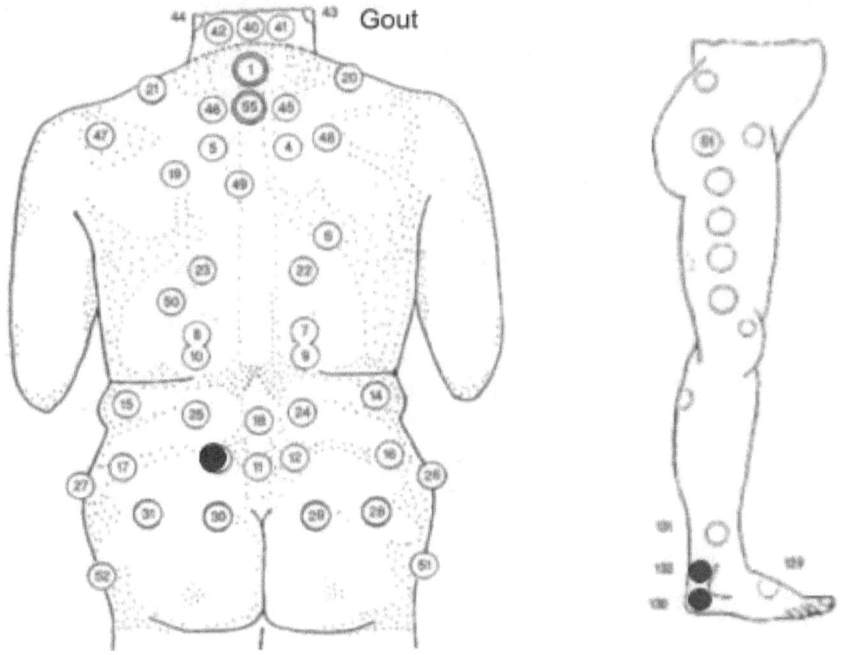

Other gout treatments

Your diet is very important when it comes to preventing and treating gout. Eat less refined carbs and foods high in fat and sugar. Other high-purine foods to avoid include green beans, beer, shrimp, tofu, and alcohol. You should also reduce your salt intake. Drink more water and eat more vegetables like potatoes and fruit, especially citrus fruit and watermelon. Ermiao wan, meadow saffron, and dandelion have all been shown to help reduce the acids that cause gout. They also reduce inflammation and pain.

Cupping and weight loss

In Traditional Chinese Medicine, weight gain is caused by a stagnant "qi" or "life energy," which can be described as poor blood flow. Stimulating certain acupressure points by cupping along the lymphatic lines of the body gets that blood flow going again. The "lymphatic lines" refers to the circulatory and immune system. By activating energy in your circulatory and immune system, the body is better equipped to metabolize bad fat. The cupping also helps relieve stress, removes toxins, and stimulates the digestive system. Cupping is never the only method patients use for weight loss - it will only help if the patient is exercising and eating well.

Unlike with basic dry cupping, cupping for weight loss requires more movement from the cups. The cups essentially "glide" over the body while maintaining a vacuum seal. The cups should move along your "problem" areas in addition to the lymphatic lines. The lymphatic system is responsible for removing toxins and waste from the body, so stimulating that helps get rid of junk. In the image on the next page, you can see the tissues and organs involved, and how the lines are organized.

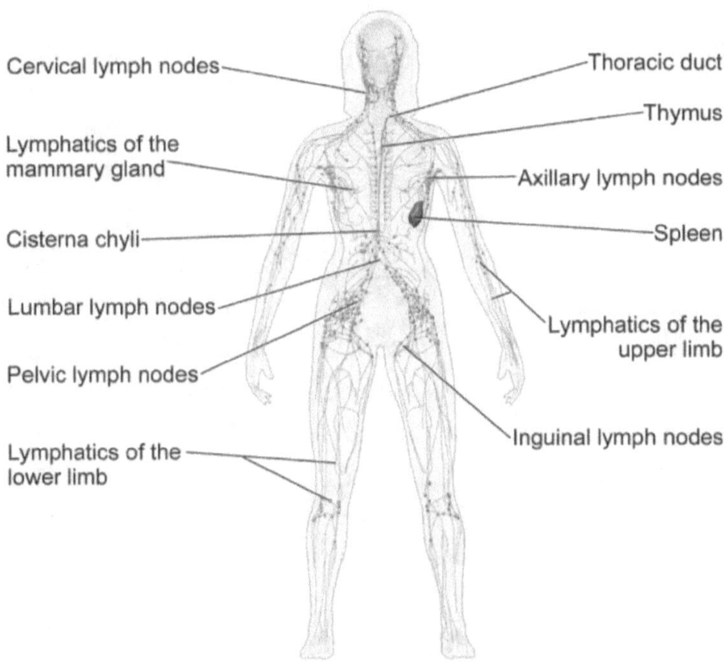

Electroacupuncture can also help with weight loss. The device generating the low current of electricity stimulates the target area for 30 minutes. This encourages the breakdown of fat. Then, normal flash and/or massage cupping is performed.

Buttocks

Toning on the buttocks is a common request for cosmetic cupping. Just one silicone cup is needed, and the therapist should apply lots of oil. Medium-strength cupping is usually okay, and after a few sessions, strong cupping can be applied. There are two ways to massage this area. The first has the therapist begin on the outside of the buttocks and moving the cup up towards the upper thigh, and then right over the buttock's main muscle (the gluteus maximus). The therapist stops once the cup reaches the lower back. The other technique starts at the middle of the flank, which is where a person's "love handles" are. Move across the buttocks muscle sideway towards the hip joint. A toning massage for the buttocks usually lasts 5-10 minutes for the first time.

Cellulite

80-90% of women have cellulite, which resembles cottage cheese, and it can be caused by genetics as well as weight gain. It actually doesn't necessary mean "fat." According to Traditional Chinese Medicine, it's caused by poor lymphatic circulation which causes lipid build-up beneath the skin. Cupping increases blood flow and gets those lipids moving. It can take 3 months of cupping treatment for a patient to notice a difference. Exercise and sufficient hydration help speed up the process.

Cupping for cellulite occurs most commonly on the upper leg and buttocks. For those areas, you'll start with the back of the body first. Oil the leg all the way from the ankles to the hip. The therapist should massage the area with their hands first to warm it up. Light cupping and flash-cupping should be applied first for just 10 minutes. As treatments continue, cupping can be strengthened and the time extended. The therapist begins cupping at the back of the lower leg and moves up towards the thigh and buttocks. For the front of the body, oil from the knee up to the groin, and start cupping at the knee and work up.

Other treatments for weight loss/toning

Our society offers a lot of ways to lose weight and tone muscle, but most of them don't work. In Traditional Chinese

Medicine, getting to (and maintaining) a healthy weight is all about mindfulness and enhancing one's qi. There aren't shortcuts or starvation diets involved. Eat whole foods full of qi, such as fresh vegetables, whole grains, and organic meat. Refined, packaged foods are terrible for the body, as is sugar and too much alcohol.

A regular eating schedule is also essential, with 7am-9am being the best time for digestion. Light dinners are recommended at around 5pm. When you eat, avoid distractions and take your time. A 10:30pm bedtime is best, as the liver cleans the blood between 1-3am, and you want to be in a deep sleep when that happens.

For herbs, there are quite a few that can make weight loss easier. Ginseng increases your metabolism, so you store less fat, and it boosts your energy. The Pu-erh herb stimulates the spleen, allowing it to better absorb and digest, and eliminate waste. You can drink it as a tea. It also increases metabolism. Guggul, which is a tree resin stabilizes and increases metabolism, and helps regulate the excretory system.

Treating skin problems

Issues with one's skin are caused by a myriad of factors, including diet, personal hygiene, genetics, and age. Today's society often recommends harsh cleansers and fancy tools, but Traditional Chinese Medicine seeks to draw out the problems from within. Cupping as a form of skincare has become increasingly popular over the years. Both facial cupping and cupping on the back are common treatments. Facial cupping is not done directly on existing acne, though it can be used to reduce the presence of scars. Cupping can also reduce the appearance of stretch marks.

Scars/stretch marks

When suction is applied to the scar tissue, it pulls it apart, allowing new blood to circulate and heal. Cupping works best with new scars. Many surgeons have found that vacuum cupping helps with post-surgery skin concerns, like integrating skin grafts and scarring from cosmetic surgery.

To perform cupping for a scar, treat the area with oil. Apply a light suction, especially if the scar is on the face, and glide the cup around on all sides of the scar. Horizontal and zigzag movements are all good. Like with standard cupping, each session should only go on for 5-10 minutes. After the cup has been removed, the scar tissue should be lightened. Stretch marks are treated with the same method.

Existing acne/cystic acne

To treat acne, cupping is done on the back at certain points, which you can find by looking at the graph and labels. Generally, cupping isn't performed directly on acne on the face, because that causes it to pop, which can lead to infection and scarring. Instead, therapists target points that correspond to issues that cause acne, and by cupping, inflammation and toxins are removed. However, you *can* cup on acne on other parts of the body. If the acne breaks, disinfect the wound with 75% alcohol.

For cupping high up on the back, right under the neck, a therapist retains the cup for 10-15 minutes. For the middle and lower back, massage cupping is applied.

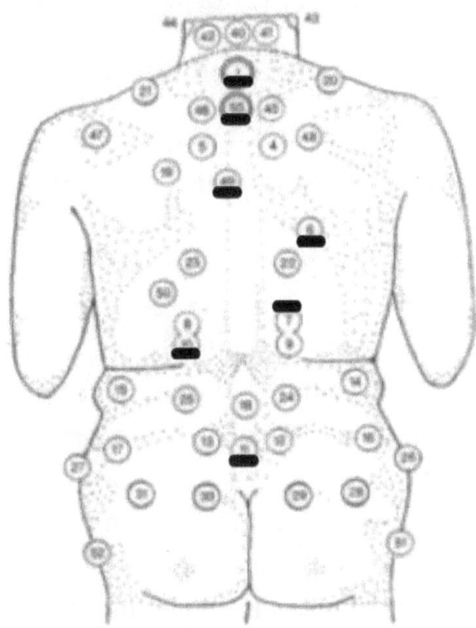

There's also a point on the leg that can be cupped for 10-15 minutes. It's found about a thumb's width from the knee on the inner part of the leg.

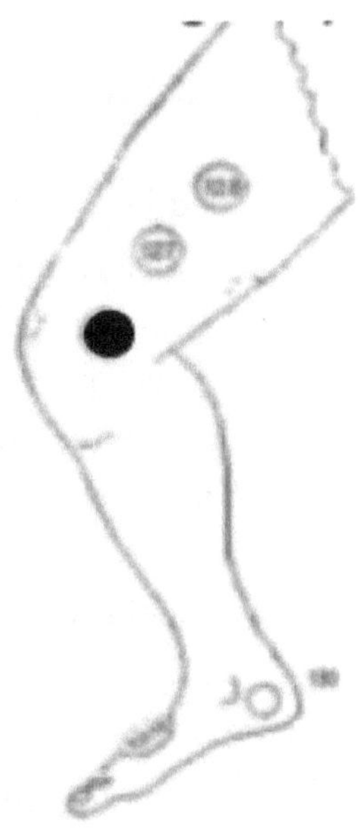

General facial skincare

For an overall healthier glow on your face, facial cupping can be performed. There are a lot of benefits to this type of treatment, including stimulated collagen production, less puffiness and redness, and pores that appear smaller. You want to cup on a completely clean face. Apply oil and massage the neck, face, and collar bone to warm up the skin. Remember, as with all facial cupping, you want special small cups and you aren't going to apply a strong suction. Facial cupping should never produce bruises, but the skin will be light pink. You should *not* cup over moles.

Place cup on face and apply a light suction. Move the cup around, using the smallest one for underneath the eyes and eyebrows, on the nose, and around your mouth. You can use a slightly-bigger one for your forehead, jaw, and cheeks. When you're first trying this type of cupping, stick to 5 minutes at first. Remove cups and wash your face to remove the oil. You should see a pronounced difference in your skin after six treatments.

Cupping over a boil or abscess

This type of cupping could be messier, and requires you to wear surgical gloves. It's a bit risky, too, since your skin will actually open. You want to be extra-sure to have clean hands, skin, and tools. Choose a wider cup, since ones with narrow lids can be very painful. Proceed with the process as normal; you don't need to use oil, since you aren't moving the cup around. Apply the cup over the boil and squeeze to create the suction. You don't actually want to try to pop the boil. What the cupping does is encourage blood flow to the area and speed up the healing process. However, the boil might pop because of the suction. If this happens, you want to clean the area and bandage it, like you would a wound.

Other treatments for skin issues

If you're dealing with acne, avoid washing your face with strong irritants. For example, skin cleansers designed for oily skin are often too harsh, and remove too much oil. Avoid fragrances, sodium lauryl sulfate, and alcohols. In terms of diet, avoid spicy food, cow's milk, sugar, and junk food. Eat more dark leafy greens, berries, and zinc-rich foods like pumpkin seeds.

For eczema or rashes, it's best to avoid washing the area more than absolutely necessary, since this irritates it further. You can also eat foods like green beans, cucumber, and lettuce, which clear heat from the body. Eat less fish, garlic, pepper, beef, and shrimp. The best thing you can do for any skin problem is to drink more water. Consuming herbs like burdock, angelica, white peony, and tribulus nourish and detoxify the skin from the inside out.

Improving hair quality

If your hair is flat, lifeless, or graying before it's time, it indicates a more serious health problem. In Traditional Chinese Medicine, your hair health reflects your kidneys and the level of blood and other fluids in your body. Having dull, lifeless, or prematurely-gray hair suggests a possible kidney and blood deficiency. To remedy that, cupping is performed on the back, bottom of the foot, and leg.

The point on the foot has been used before, and it's often referred to as the "gushing spring" point. It's the Kidney 1 (K1) pressure point, so it addresses a kidney deficiency head on. The other points are found in the leg, right next to and above the ankle, and by the knee. A therapist will knead the points first, perform cupping for 10-15 minutes, and then use moxibustion for 3-5 minutes. The points on the back provide nourishment to the blood. Retain suction for 10-15 minutes.

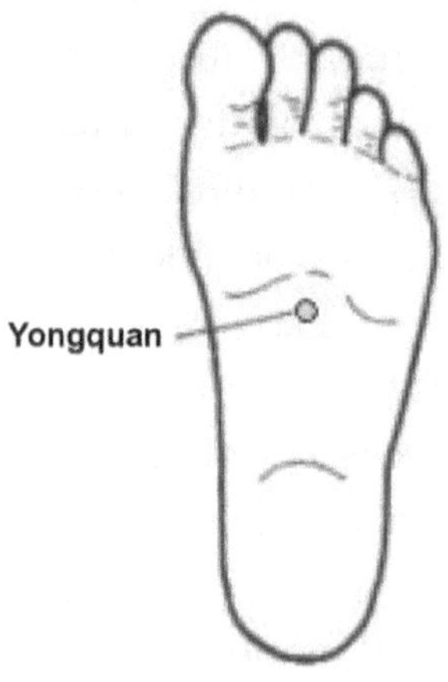

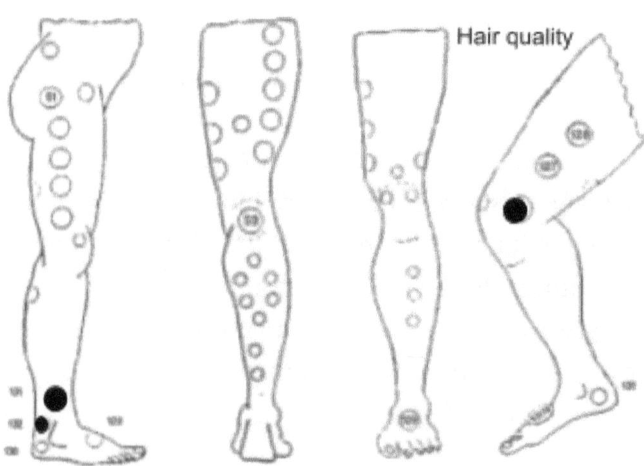

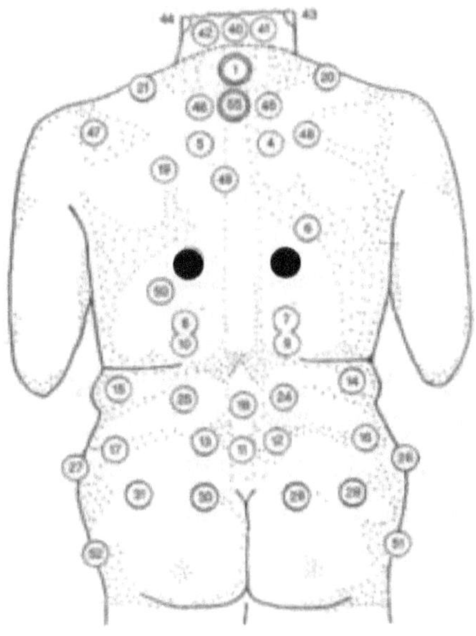

Other treatments for healthier hair

Treating your hair should start from the inside out. A change in diet can have a positive impact, so eat more foods rich in folic acid, which restores red blood cells. Spinach and lentils are both high in folic acid. You can also eat tangerines, salmon, and Greek yogurt to prevent hair loss. Sweet potatoes help moisten dry hair.

For herbs, fallopia is very popular. It strengthens the kidney meridian and nourishes the blood. Rehmannia has also shown promise in preventing premature graying, while Dong Quai ("female ginseng") can treat split ends, dryness, and brittle hair.

When is it safe to try cupping at home?

I've stated multiple times that most professionals agree cupping should only be performed by a licensed therapist. However, if you are going to try cupping at home, you should follow the general rule that treating something external is safer than something internal. That means if your health concern is superficial and involves an issue on the outside or close to the outside of your body (i.e. scars, acne, weight loss), it's relatively safe to try and treat it yourself. However, the further inside the body you go, you start dealing with organs and bodily functions. There may be a more serious problem going on that you don't recognize. Those issues require more skill and knowledge, so a professional should be entrusted with treatment.

C h a p t e r   6

What to Remember

There's a lot of information out there on cupping and its possible health effects, and it can be hard to know what to take away from all of it. This chapter summarizes what we covered and provides some key takeaways to remember before you attempt cupping with a professional or at home.

The science on cupping isn't solid

The majority of doctors agree that the benefits of cupping (dry or wet) are not supported by science. The main reason is that there simply aren't enough studies that allow the medical community to form any kind of consensus. Because of the nature of science, nothing is ever "settled," but when a sufficient of evidence exists for one side or the other, scientists can make statements with more certainty. For example, acupuncture is still considered by many to be a pseudoscience, but there's been a lot of research and solid evidence to suggest that it can work to relieve chronic pain. It's important to know where a medical therapy stands with the scientific community, so you can stay informed and safe.

Know the risks

Speaking of staying safe, cupping has risks you should remember before seeking out the therapy. Traditional dry cupping that uses flame can cause burns and inflammation, while both fire and vacuum cupping can cause blood clots. Wet cupping is the riskiest form, because cutting the skin can lead to infection. Cupping as a replacement for other treatment can have potentially fatal consequences if you are treating an illness like cancer or diabetes. If you plan on trying cupping treatment, you should also be aware that doing any form at home without a professional significantly increases the risks, and most resources urge people against DIY therapy.

Know what to ask a doctor/therapist

Cupping is often touted as a therapy that's great for everyone, but that isn't necessarily true. Before receiving treatment, you should talk to your doctor and a cupping therapist. Some questions to ask include:

- Am I receiving the standard treatments for my health concern?
- Are there any reasons why I shouldn't try cupping?
- What is your training?
- How experienced are you with cupping?
- When would you recommend cupping?

If trying cupping at home, be extra careful about meeting hygiene standards

If you do try cupping at home, there are certain guidelines you should always meet. You can't be *too* clean. Always sterilize your cups before and after use. Always cup in a clean area and use clean towels. When it comes to caring for the body, you want to perform cupping on clean skin. If you think you're being too careful, you aren't.

Know how to cup in a way that results in as little pain as possible

The phrase "No pain, no gain" does *not* apply to cupping. While you might feel discomfort during cupping, you never want to grit your teeth and fight through any pain. Everyone is different, and what is fine for one person may be too painful for someone else. Always veer on the side of light/weak suction when starting out. To make cupping as comfortable as possible, you want the cups as close to the skin as possible. That means cupping in areas with no hair. You might need to shave the area. If you're using massage cupping, always apply oil to clean skin first.

Know where (and where not to) cup

Before cupping, you should always know where you're going to place the cups. If you're cupping for pain, you want to stick to the muscle groups causing the issue, and to fleshy areas of the back, stomach, and legs. Don't put cups anywhere where you can feel a pulse, or over an artery, over deep-vein thrombosis, or on a bony area.

Adopt other healthy habits

Cupping is not a one-stop shop to health. Some people think if they receive cupping (or acupuncture), they don't have to do much else. I once knew a young woman who received acupuncture every time she had a cold, but she also refused to eat any vegetables. This type of mindset is no different than someone who just relies on pills, but doesn't take care of their body in other ways. Eat better, exercise, drink water, sleep well, and reduce stress. These healthy habits are scientifically-proven to improve your well-being. Cupping should serve as a complementary treatment; it's not a cure-all.

Epilogue

There's a lot we can learn from the ancient past. In East Asia and places like Egypt and Iraq, doctors practiced a variety of techniques to treat chronic pain and illnesses. One of those techniques - cupping - has been making a comeback thanks to exposure from athletes and celebrities. Through the power of suction on different points on the body, cupping encourages healthy blood flow, removes toxins, and encourages the body to perform its functions more effectively.

In this book, we covered the different types of cupping, including traditional dry cupping, which uses glass cups and heat to generate suction. In more recent times, vacuum cupping has become common, which gets rid of heat and replaces glass with flexible plastic, rubber, and silicone cups. This allows therapists to move the cups around on the body more easily for massage cupping. Because of the availability of cupping kits, people are trying cupping at home, which does have risks. At-home cupping isn't recommended by professionals. There are also certain people who shouldn't receive cupping at all, like those with a pacemaker, a fever, or a bleeding illness like hemophilia.

What can dry cupping treat? Historically, cupping has been used to treat every kind of health problem. Headaches, digestion issues, skin issues, diabetes, and congestion can all improve with cupping on specific points on the body. This book included charts to show the location of the relevant points.

Scientific research on cupping is limited, so doctors cannot say for sure whether the reported benefits of cupping are accurate. Like acupuncture, the effects of cupping may be a combination of a placebo and actual medical value. Before receiving a cupping treatment, you should talk to your doctor and do further research on any risks. While many agree that cupping is safe, there are risks and certain people should not receive the treatment. Regardless of whether cupping truly works or not, you should set realistic expectations and be healthy in other ways. Cupping can be a part of a healthy lifestyle, but it isn't a miracle cure for any health condition.